THE
FRAGRANT
YEAR

৯০

THE FRAGRANT YEAR

*Seasonal Meditations with
Aromatherapy Oils*

JANE GRAYSON

Illustrated by Claire Hedges

Aquarian/Thorsons
An Imprint of HarperCollins*Publishers*

The Aquarian Press
An Imprint of HarperCollins*Publishers*
77–85 Fulham Palace Road,
Hammersmith, London W6 8JB
1160 Battery Street,
San Francisco, California 94111-1213

Published by The Aquarian Press 1993

1 3 5 7 9 10 8 6 4 2

©Jane Grayson 1993

Jane Grayson asserts the moral right to
be identified as the author of this work
A catalogue record for this book
is available from the British Library

ISBN 0 7225 2863 9

Printed by HarperCollinsManufacturing,
Hong Kong

CONTENTS

To Evelyn

But flowers distilled,
though they with winter meet,
Lose but their show;
their substance still lives sweet.

William Shakespeare, from Sonnet 5

INTRODUCTION

A perfume, a piece of music, a poem or a beautiful painting, all have the power to charm, to change a mood, to transport us momentarily from our mundane world into a more fanciful existence. Unlike words or images, however, a perfume speaks to the most primeval of the senses, that of smell, and this gives it a special quality all of its own. Unseen, unheard, it creeps across boundaries and touches the soul at the deepest, most instinctive level.

Chemists never seem to tire of playing with them, but even they often admit that perfumes have a mind of their own and their appeal is a very personal one. Synthetic or otherwise, we all have our favourites, but Nature's delicate scents play a far more important role in our lives than perhaps we realize.

Smell affects the ancient seat of the brain in much the same way as light and heat. These messages trigger responses in animals for mating and hibernation and in man the delicate hormonal balance can be tipped in a similar fashion. As the air is full of colour, sound and scent, the subtle energy centres in the body open and, like the flowers themselves, respond to the language of the natural world.

Wind-pollinated plants such as grasses have little scent or colour, for they do not need it, but the brightness of many flowers attracts insects and bees from a distance. Then, as they draw closer, they pick up the scent. A bee's olfactory receptors are in its feelers, so as it smells it is also feeling and examining. Surprisingly, a similar connection has been suggested in the human nose.

It seems that tiny sense organs in our own noses respond to the microscopic 'shapes' that make up the molecules of scents. With a locking mechanism, our senses relate to the geometry of odours and this is how we discriminate between them.

During the summer months the air is full of magic as herbs and flowers release their fragrant essences into the atmosphere – who has not lingered with the scent of roses after a shower of rain? Mankind's efforts to extract these exquisite entities have resulted in various aromatic substances being produced since the beginning of time. However, it was not until the perfection of distillation that he was able to capture the pure, unadulterated essence of the plant – the so-called 'essential oil'.

Originally, these precious substances were handled only by experienced physicians, but in time they were bottled, marketed and travelled the trade routes carrying their lovely messages across cultural barriers. Ripening like wine, now they could keep for far longer periods.

'A liquid prisoner pent in walls of glass': Shakespeare's description of an essential oil some 400 years after the first one had been produced in the Middle East. Distillation probably originated in China where it was the domain of the so-called 'alchemists'. They practised their art with a ritualistic precision that was in strict accordance with the interplay of light and dark and other natural rhythms that effect plant life, especially that of the moon.

The sun's is a logical, predictable force, but the moon is more mysterious, waxing and waning and moving about the sky, sometimes leaving her shadow there until late in the day, sometimes disappearing altogether. In winter her magnetic power is vital, moving the tides of subterranean waters and favouring germinating seeds underground.

Natural fragrances have a moonlike quality, they can be unpredictable and are intimately connected with the subconscious mind. Like a reflection in a pool, they put us in touch with the person we know is there, but somehow cannot quite reach.

> Even the seasons form a great circle in their changing,
> and always come back again to where they were. The life
> of a man is a circle from childhood to childhood and so it
> is in everything where power moves.
>
> Black Elk, *Holy Man of the Oglala Sioux*, 1931

Our remote ancestors understood natural cycles and their lives were an integral part of the fluctuating drama of the natural world. They understood its language and spoke to it through the rhythm of drums, their songs, colour, imagery and perfume, often in the form of incense.

The medium for getting in touch with this world was usually a wise member of the tribe, but at certain times of the year the fine curtain between the seen and the unseen was more easily lifted by the ordinary person. This was especially true at the changing seasons and gradually, as people became more agricultural and settled, these times were marked by established festivals, some of which are still observed today.

In Britain, the original 'calendar' was an acknowledgement of the 28-day cycle of the moon. This was changed, first by the conquering Romans, and later to the Gregorian calendar which we still use today. The natural world, however, does not live by diaries and filofaxes; we may add a day here and there, but the moon's cycle remains unchanged, the seasons shift and the wheel of the zodiac turns, all without any help from us. My book is an acknowledgement of this natural rhythm.

Most of the festivals referred to in this book are of Celtic origin, but the beliefs and practices of the Celts are echoed in many other cultures, for our ancient links are surprisingly strong.

We, too, are part of nature and respond to the pull of her magnetic force, especially in the tides of our subconscious where ancestral memories are lodged. Now, more than ever, this is suppressed and submerged in the rush of modern life.

Much of our knowledge of plants and flowers is handed down from remote times and cultures all over the globe as part of our heritage. Herbs, flowers, trees, still respond to ancient rhythms and play a valuable role in allowing us to rediscover a more natural pattern to life.

This book is my own personal interpretation of the power of essential oils. It invites you on a fragrant journey through the year in the company of some of the loveliest natural perfumes. Against a backdrop of the changing seasons their characters are brought to life, but they can be used at any time of the year when their particular qualities are most needed. The seasons themselves reflect the cycle of the Northern Hemisphere, but this can easily be adjusted to suit any part of the world.

Through the beautiful medium of essential oils, herbs and flowers, together with simple meditations and visualizations, it is hoped you will find something to help with the ups and downs of life. Essential oils are volatile, they evaporate easily. *Volare* means to fly in Latin and indeed they do. On gossamer wings they will transport you to other worlds, open up new vistas of awareness and help you to establish a better balance in life.

Inhale them for short periods only and do not apply them to the skin unless you have received guidance from a properly trained aromatherapist. Methods of extraction tend to dictate the terminology applied to essential oils. For the sake of convenience, however, the word 'essence' has been used in most cases throughout the book.

*B*REATH

This is not a book about breathing, but it goes without saying that if you are inhaling a perfume then the rhythm of your breath is very important. The air we breathe is central to our existence. We can go a fair while without food and water, but only a few minutes without air. When a baby is born the most important thing is to ensure the first breath: once that has been drawn a new life on this earth has begun. Everything in the universe breathes and in Chinese medicine, the vital *Chi* energy that runs through every living thing has been translated as 'breath'.

The Persian physician, Avicenna, thought to have produced the first pure, distilled essence of Rose, believed that the divine, universal force was drawn into the body by the breath. For him that 'breath of life' was closely linked to the heart, the organ most susceptible to emotional changes in a person. He advocated the use of natural perfumes as a way of treating diseases of the heart and regulating breathing.

Most urban city dwellers are very shallow breathers. There is little fresh air available and the pace of modern life can create fears and agitations that make respiration ever faster and more erratic.

If you do the little exercises in this book, always be aware of the ebb and flow of your breath. Do not become obsessed by it, but simply let it be steady and regular as you inhale the beautiful fragrances. For those interested in taking it further, the art of breathing can be taught through the practice of yoga and similar disciplines.

FRAGRANCE BURNERS

These usually consist of an attractive ceramic or stoneware stand which supports a small bowl or container of water with a small candle underneath. Put a couple of drops of essential oil into the water and light the candle. The heat will vaporize the essence into the atmosphere. Fragrance burners are the most appropriate for a meditation. A simple substitute is to put a few drops of essence into a bowl of hot water.

DIFFUSERS OR NEBULIZERS

Good versions of these actually pump the aromatic molecules into the atmosphere – excellent for dealing with airborne germs. They are usually made of glass and comprise a bowl which takes a small amount of neat essential oil – no water is used – a little chamber which disperses the molecules into a fine mist, and an electric pump. Several versions exist for home and therapy use, although some can be noisy.

Other versions make use of a stable electronic plate onto which a couple of drops of essential oil are placed. The heated plate vaporizes the fragrance quickly into the atmosphere, but does not pump it out in the same way as the glass versions. This type is usually very quiet.

VAPORIZING RING

A ceramic ring which is placed round a light bulb, when the light is switched on, the heat generates the fragrance.

SMELLING STRIPS

Thin strips of absorbent paper, a useful alternative to sniffing straight from the bottle. Just one drop on the end of the strip is usually sufficient. Wave under the nose or place in a small vase or container on a table in front of you.

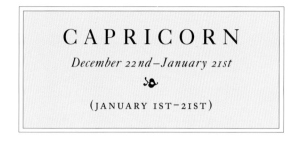

CAPRICORN

December 22nd–January 21st

ॐ

(JANUARY 1ST–21ST)

In the month of January, the first of the series, God makes us into hermits. God has whitewashed the black earth all around; there is no underwood without its white dress, there is no copse without its coverlet.

Dafydd ap Gwilym, *The Snow*, 14th Century

The Celts called the period between December and January 'cold time' and 'stay home time'. These dark months called for withdrawal and regeneration, in keeping with the natural cycle, and other cultures agreed with them. The *Nei Ching*, an ancient Chinese medical text, describes this as a time when 'all things in creation live shut in and the crop is stored away' and advises us to 'compress and conceal our wishes'.

Now the Sun's influence is weak, but the Moon's magnetism is strong, especially underground where a new cycle of life has already begun. Now, in the raw half light of a cold January morning, while Nature sleeps, we make our New Year resolutions. Some may last no more than a day, but behind these brave resolves lies a subconscious belief in the continuing cycle of life. Although we make them now, they are still frozen in time, it will take the year's turning to bring them to fruition.

NEW YEAR'S DAY

> And Hezekiah hearkened unto them, and shewed them
> all the house of his precious things, the silver, and the
> gold, and the spices. . .   II Kings 20:13

Most New Year's Resolutions are made in a spirit of health and wealth, together with traditional spicy fare. Gifts from the East, our festive spices began to arrive in Britain in the 11th and 12th Centuries. Cinnamon, cloves, nutmeg, saffron and many more commanded such high prices that they changed the destinies of nations. In Britain the Guild of Pepperers was set up to deal with the entire range of spices and perfumes and the term 'peppercorn rent' indicates that all these precious commodities frequently changed hands instead of money.

CLOVE BUD (*Eugenia caryophyllata*)*
Clove was especially valued and its original source, the tropical 'spice islands' was a closely guarded secret.

Cloves themselves are the unopened flower buds which are picked and left in the hot sun to dry. Rich pickings indeed. Examine one. You are holding a tiny powerhouse of tropical energy. Entire economies were transformed by these little 'nails' as the French called them.

Hold a few in your palm. See them rolling like dice through the hands of wealthy Renaissance merchants, or packed on cargo ships alongside silks, satins and other treasures. Then crush and inhale them.

Clove has a fragrance full of riches. A fiery heat laced with velvet. From its rich base comes a fruity, satisfying note. Clove really is the classic spice.

As a bringer of wealth and stability to nations, Clove carries a strongly protective aura, but greater and older by far is its reputation as a healer. In the heat of its native land, the trees released their antiseptic perfume into the air, keeping the people free from fevers. In Europe, Clove soon became an important panacea during the epidemics and pandemics which followed in the wake of the very trade that brought it here.

With a colourful past at the extreme end of wealth and disease, Clove has no illusions about life and combines endurance with a ruthless determination when necessary. It will dispel any wariness or guilt over money and is the supreme optimist. Why have a silver lining when gold is available? It has the scent of magic, but knows all the pitfalls, and its domain is the here and now. It is ideal for a meditation on New Year's Day.

---

[*] A beautiful essence of Clove is available, but should only be applied to the skin by someone who is properly qualified.

CLOVE: MEDITATION

This meditation is concerned with material wealth, but if you do not like this idea apply it to any personal desire or attachment.

Are you being honest about your attitude towards money and possessions? There is a difference between clinging to material wealth and simply enjoying it. To let go of attachment can be a way of attracting more good things into your life.

Sit by a table and on it place something that you are particularly fond of, a piece of jewellery or an ornament.

Breathe in:	Hold your breath for a moment and as you do,
	hold the love that you have for that object.
Breathe out:	Gently release your breath and with it give
	that love away to the Universe.
Open your eyes:	The object is still there,
	but the Universe is grateful.

Try the exercise again. This time be aware of the fragrance of Clove. Draw in that rich, fulfilling scent. Clove knows the texture of gold and can bring it into your life, but can you handle it responsibly?

The gift of Love is golden.

ORANGE *(Citrus aurantium sinensis)**
The fruity note in Clove calls to Orange to temper its force.

Both arrived here at roughly the same time and have enjoyed a successful working relationship ever since; they complement each other beautifully. A well-known example is the original pomander – an orange stuck with cloves.

Orange brings a softness to their relationship and has a warm, pleasurable appeal to the senses. Gentle and unobtrusive it makes an excellent room fragrancer, bringing a sense of ease and well-being with an antiseptic quality too. Orange is pure joy, and its sunny disposition can have quite a positive influence on the emotions, so keep it around to deal with any post-festivity blues. Not an intensely spiritual oil, but a valuable mediator which will soften any thoughts that may be becoming too arrogant.

Like other citrus oils, essence of Orange is not distilled, but pressed from the rind, and is a lovely addition to many blends.

* If applied to the skin, all the citrus oils have the potential for photosensitivity.

ORANGE AND CLOVE: NEW YEAR'S BLESSINGS MEDITATION
Clove brings good health and wealth, and Orange brings pure joy. Everything you wish for yourself and others at New Year.

Use this spirit to surround yourself with a happy, protective aura for the coming year.

Sit comfortably with a blend of Orange and Clove in the burner.

Breathe gently for a couple of minutes. As you inhale, visualize the clove groves saturating the air with their healing essence. Feel the tropical sunshine and the gentle, positive energy of orange. Both fragrances bring the sun. Surround yourself with golden light.

Breathe in: Hold this feeling there for a moment.

Breathe out: Send it out to those you love.

Capricorn Full Moon: New Beginnings Moon

If the new moon in Capricorn is early, the full moon will often fall around Twelfth Night, or Epiphany, when the early Christians in Egypt calculated the actual birthday of Christ and the three wise men were said to have presented their gifts of gold, frankincense and myrrh.

He was not the first to receive these traditional offerings to priest kings: Gold for Kingship; Frankincense for priesthood; and Myrrh to ensure resurrection after death. Myrrh appeared again after the crucifixion, brought by Nicodemus to embalm Christ's body.

In ancient Egypt the complicated embalming ritual was the supreme acknowledgement of the continuing cycle of life. The cavities of the body were often filled with 'the purest bruised Myrrh', not only because of its value as a preservative, but also for its unique perfume.

MYRRH *(Commiphora myrrha* – and other species)
Perfume was essential to Egyptian daily life. Resins continuously purified and revitalized the air, to heighten awareness and induce sleep. A perfumed, dreamlike state was an important aid in healing the sick, and in death, scent was the vital ingredient to ensure the safe passage of the soul into the next life.

> The perfume of Arabia hath been brought to thee to make perfect thy smell through the scent of the god. . . O sweet-smelling soul of the great god, thou dost contain such a sweet odour that thy face shall neither change nor perish. . .and thy soul shall appear over thy body in Ta-neter [the Divine Land].
>
> E.A. Wallis Budge, 'Incantation to Anubis', *Egyptian Magic*, 1899

To create the correct 'odour of sanctity' the priest anointed the body with sacred oils and then invoked the jackal-headed god Anubis, with his keen sense of smell, to confirm that this had been achieved. Stealing across the chasm between life and death, the scent of Myrrh was invariably present.

The essence comes from the resin and its smoky-sweet fragrance is concerned with the intimate nature of the soul. It has a lingering quality, evoking a very personal sense of trust.

Armed with thorns and spines, small and squat, yet with a dignity no cultivated plant could ever possess, Myrrh is a shaman among the desert rocks. Hermit-like, it clings to craggy surfaces, oozing resin from a thick, fragrant bark and releasing a fine, lilac incense which filters the sun's rays and protects those around it.

Sacred plant, sacred scent, mediator between worlds. Welcome, gentle transformer, to the first Full Moon of the year.

> O blest unfabled Incense Tree
> That grows in glorious Araby
> With red scent chalicing the air
> Till earth-life grow Elysian there.
>
> George Darley, 'The Phoenix', 19th Century

MYRRH: MEDITATION

Life is a process of little deaths. Each moment that ticks by, each day, each year, each cell in the body, each hair on the head, every thoughtform – each one is constantly renewing itself and always takes on a slightly different form. Human life is part of this process.

Our culture goes to a lot of trouble to erect rigid boundaries between life and death, love and sex, romance and religion. With these barriers firmly set in place, it is difficult to appreciate the ease with which a transition from one state to another can actually be made.

Most New Year Resolutions are about breaking old habits or traditions and although we may be reluctant, sooner or later we could be forced to make the adjustment anyway, especially if it is connected with our health. So let's do it now.

Whether you wish to change a relationship, or give up smoking, you will still be moving from one state into another.

Put a few drops of Myrrh into a burner, sit comfortably with one hand on each knee and visualize a beautiful deep lilac. Let the light surround you and put your hands together, as if one was shaking the other, imagine you are greeting an old friend. Squeeze them warmly and then let them go. Stretch them out in front of you. Your friend is inviting you on a journey. Breathe in the scent of Myrrh and allow the lilac to dissolve into a paler shade. Go with it and let it dissolve again into pure white light.

Make your resolution and know that you have already achieved it.

Realization is eternal.

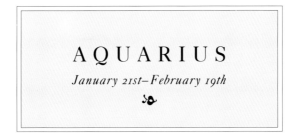

AQUARIUS

January 21st–February 19th

Thick you are, and clammy, oh father of the rain, its
homestead and its mother; a loveless crop, unsunned, a
pannier of sea coal between the sun and me, a drizzling
hurdle which brings night by day to me, a day like night
– are you not graceless?

Dafydd ap Gwilym, 'The Mist', 14th Century

Through the snow and rain, the waxing January light holds the promise
of spring, but is still bitterly cold and austere. It is important to
maintain a firm centre at this time of year.

AQUARIUS NEW MOON:
NOURISHING MOON

The waters inside the earth move up and down like a tide. The old
physicians talked of 'ground water', 'ground fire' and 'ground vapour'

being breathed in and out as though through a giant lung. In the Northern Hemisphere in late January, Earth's vapour is chilly and moist and human lungs are vulnerable. With all the festivities behind them, people can feel isolated, depleted and insular.

BENZOIN *(Styrax benzoin* – and other species)
The sweet, vanilla-like smell of Benzoin is familiar to many as a constituent of Friars Balsam. Elizabeth I loved her 'Benjamin' and had it powdered with another warm herb, Marjoram. Not surprisingly it shifts mucous and makes a wonderful inhalant. From the resin of the Styrax tree which grows in the Far East, the essence is usually thick, brown, sticky and protective. Its production is a complicated process, but the solar energy that it absorbs and conserves during this time and the care and consideration taken over its harvesting are mirrored in its effect on the human body and psyche.

Benzoin's powers of penetration are great: holding the consciousness in a velvet glove, it gently slices through inner resistance. Working on a very deep and personal level it can reveal hidden aspects of our nature. For those who have become too inward-looking and silent, its reassuring warmth creates a stable base from which to examine congealed doubts and fears and get them moving again.

Long exposure to summer sun and air gives this seemingly heavy oil a lightness that can ease communication. It creates a positive channel to the outside world, particularly when there is a need to ask for help. Draw on its strength when you are feeling low and unable to face up to life, or when an argument has drained you. Use it too when you have an important message to get across to someone, when you are far from home and wish to protect your family, or if there is someone you want to help, but simply don't know how.

BENZOIN: MEDITATION

Do this meditation in the evening, or whenever you feel you need this kind of healing energy. It is also useful if you wish to pass such energy on to someone else.

Sit quietly with a drop of Benzoin on a smelling strip and simply linger with the fragrance.

Breathe deeply and imagine you are in tune with the great lungs of the earth. Find a steady rhythm that you are comfortable with and settle into it.

Allow the fragrance to seep into your senses carrying its healing force right down into your feet. Feel the warmth of its loving nature, your senses are wrapped in a warm, brown velvet. You can trust it, let it do its own work.

Now draw that warmth and energy back up into your chest. Breathe gently as you hold it there, nurturing it. Then take a deep breath and let it go.

Everyone needs to be healed, even healers themselves. It is
OK to ask for help.

*I*MBOLG: THE RETURN OF THE GODDESS:
JANUARY 31ST

The Snowdrop
Many, many welcomes
February fair-maid
Ever as of old time,
Solitary firstling,
Coming in the cold time,
Prophet of the gay time,
Prophet of the May time,
Prophet of the roses,
Many, many welcomes
February fair-maid!

Alfred Lord Tennyson, 19th Century

The snowdrop symbolized the return of Brigid, the Moon Goddess. As she carpeted the Druid's groves, Celtic women gathered to welcome her. Clothed in white with all the purity and innocence of new life, she emerged to bestow her blessings. From now until Hallowe'en, her magnetic power would no longer be hidden.

Ushered in by the new moon in Aquarius, the influence of this lovely festival lasted through to the Spring Equinox. Echoes of it can be heard in the myths of the Egyptian goddess, Isis, the Greek Persephone,

Demeter, and many others. For us it became St Bride's Day and later Candlemass, dedicated to the Virgin Mary.

Women dressed in white carried candles and performed rituals at holy wells and springs. Wearing shiny ornaments, reminiscent of flowing water, in the bitter cold they fanned the flames of fires to encourage the flow of their own life-giving essences as well as those of their animals and of the rivers and streams.

The breaking and flow of waters was at the heart of this festival. The lactation of ewes and subsequent birth of lambs promised milk and cheese for the diet and a quickening, not only of the senses, but also of the fluids of the body. Storage and regeneration were giving way to purification, cleansing and renewed energy.

This is still a time of powerful transformation when all of Nature's alchemy is at work, slowly drawing back the Light. Cushioned by technology, we can ignore its passing, but on grey February days, its spirit stirs the lonely sea of the subconscious where modern illusions dissolve. A reminder, in this world of reservoirs, radiators and incubators, that life's most basic needs have changed little. A fresh supply of clear water, a safe passage for the newborn into this world and above all, a fertile earth.

> And thou shalt have goat's milk enough for thy food, for the food of thy household, and for the maintenance of thy maidens.
>
> Proverbs 27:26

29

ROSEMARY (*Rosemarinus officinalis*)

> Rosemary comforteth the braine, the memorie,
> and the inward senses and restoreth speech unto
> them that are possessed with the dumb palsie.
>
> John Gerard, *The History of Plants*, 1597

Called 'evermore green', Rosemary loves the sun, but is not dependent on its rhythm. Its silver-green leaves breathe all year round and give up their essence willingly, even in winter. Brush them in December and smell your fingers – what a gift this plant is! Its reputation for keeping the memory fresh probably comes from this evergreen quality.

'It is an holy tree and with folk that be just and rightfull gladlye it groweth and thryveth', wrote a clerk of the School of Salerno in 1338. Never far from the people, this apothecary among plants sacrifices its flower power to produce intensely aromatic leaves rich in medicinal essence. Tiny, but of the palest blue, its flowers were once thought to have been white, but in keeping with its chaste reputation were changed by the touch of the Virgin Mary.

By stimulating the circulation of oxygen in the body, Rosemary tones the heart, helps the flow of blood to the brain, and benefits that master detoxifier, the liver. Old herbals tell us it is for 'keeping the breath sweet' and it can also help us to prevent adversity from turning us sour.

Rosemarinus 'Rose of the Sea', this plant's affinity for water is concerned with flow and return, shifting stagnant moisture and turning the emotional tide. This natural recycler encourages us to be economical with our energy and to distance ourselves from emotional pulls without losing compassion. Not a romantic or seductive oil, but one which helps to build on existing relationships.

Rosemary's circular action stimulates and eases restriction, but at this quickening time of year, makes sure nothing breaks too soon. Like all things, if it is born too early, the force will be weak and malformed.

ROSEMARY: MEDITATION

Best done in the morning.

Life's lessons are circular, they keep coming round again and again until we have understood them. The natural element governing the spirit of Imbolg is Water. It can be fresh and flowing or stale and stagnant. Have you ever noticed familiar patterns manifesting in your life? The way you react when you are on the defensive perhaps, or always choosing the same type of mate and ending up with the same old hurt?

When we do acknowledge these things, our reactions can be circular too. We can get conveniently busy, racing about, doing anything rather than face up to them. The trouble is, it's the same old stagnant water going round and round.

Rosemary's bright, uplifting scent is sweet and penetrating. Its invigorating energy will revitalize your own and is especially useful if you are simply feeling tired or liverish.

Sit near a window in the light. Have some Rosemary in a fragrance burner, or you could hold a sprig of the herb.

Inhale the fragrance and as you do so, you will feel its clean, refreshing light flowing through your senses, especially your head. Acknowledge its circular action.

As you breathe in, see this fluid energy circulating as a soft, silver green, then let it change to the palest blue or aquamarine. As you breathe out, let it change to white.

Fresh energy is vital, life is a process of renewal.

$\mathcal{A}$QUARIUS FULL MOON:
MOON OF PURITY

With its mists and vapours and weakly-growing sunshine, this fluid time of year can bring a sense of the unseen uncannily close, leaving us melancholy and moody. The purifying forces of Nature are hard at work, but in the stillness of a late February day, as melting ice reveals the sludge underneath, it is easy for submerged fears and anxieties to come floating to the surface of the conscious mind.

JUNIPER BERRY (*Juniperus communis*)

Juniper has the power to flush out unwanted emotions very quickly; its sharp, piquant scent is full of hot vitality.

The beautiful blue-black berries are resinous and aromatic and have been found between the bandages of Egyptian mummies. The fragrant branches burn with a pure, bright light and have been a favourite for purification ceremonies for centuries. Such rituals were important after the close confinement of winter as communities prepared for a lighter and more energetic way of life.

While Rosemary's action is circular, Juniper's is concerned with the outward expression of purity and flow. Its fiery quality can dispel congealed emotions and dissolve any crystalline conditions lingering in the psyche.

If you have suffered a deep loss and are depleted or weepy, it will speed your recovery. If this experience is really blocking your progress, combine it with Myrrh. The exquisite, bitter-sweet quality of this blend will bring a sympathy to your suffering, especially if you are using the pain negatively to prevent life from moving on.

To shake off bad vibrations and clear the brain of clutter, rub a drop of Juniper between your palms and brush it through your hair. Feel its silver fluidity washing your senses clean. Or put some in a burner to cleanse the atmosphere in a room. You can even burn a few berries on some charcoal.

JUNIPER: MEDITATION

This meditation is best done in the morning.

Put a few drops of Juniper in a fragrance burner and sit facing the light.

As you breathe visualize a glistening current flowing straight through you, flushing your system clean.

Think of an icicle melting. As the sun's rays get stronger, it starts to flow and gradually it becomes a silver stream. The stream is flowing between high banks of snow, but as it travels the snow too starts to melt, revealing grassy green banks. There is nothing you can do to stop it, and why should you anyway, it is beautiful. If you feel like it, get in and let the clear water wash over you. The fluid quality of turquoise and silver is good for a colour visualization.

Life is moving. Go with the flow.

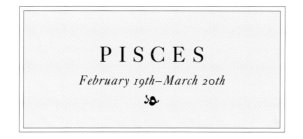

PISCES

February 19th–March 20th

Subtle and secretive, the etheric waters of Pisces are watched over by the Moon, but moved towards a greater creativity by Jupiter. As the silvery new moon waxes, the fruits of that gentle energy start to appear.

$\mathcal{P}$*ISCES NEW MOON:*
MOON OF FIRST FULFILMENT

A Contemplation upon Flowers
You are not proud, you know your birth
For your embroider'd garments are from Earth:

You do obey your months, but I
Would have it ever spring.

My fate would know no winter, never die
Nor think of such a thing.

Henry King, 'A Contemplation Upon Flowers', 17th Century

SPRING FLOWERS

How does one define these elusive scents of early spring? With no warm breeze to waft them they hang low on the cold air and take us by surprise.

Crocus, daffodil, narcissus, hyacinth, all the pastel shades appear as the pure white of the Snowdrop starts to fade. Relatives of the Lily and with the same feminine quality, their waxy delicacy is often surrounded by ice and snow. How do they survive? What is their secret? These early flowers have no need of us. They are true representatives of the Underworld, where streams and rivers still flow, and safe in their womb-like bulbs they carry their own water supply. Now the full moon of Pisces, house of secrets, reveals her hidden treasures. Serene and untroubled by their surroundings, these flowers are a tranquil moment in time. They give us space to pause, take a deep breath and drink their fragrance before the onrush of spring.

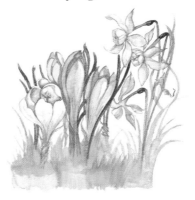

And in the moment betwixt the breathing in
And the breathing out
Is hidden all the mysteries
Of the Infinite Garden.

Edmond Bordeaux Szekely, 'Communions',
The Essene Gospel of Peace, Book Two

Very few essential oils are available from these flowers. Those that are, though beautiful, are very expensive. The scent of Narcissus can sometimes be slightly narcotic, even in the flower.

SPRING FLOWERS: MEDITATION

The haunting fragrance of a hyacinth, or a pot of narcissus is ideal for this, but a vase of spring flowers will do just as well. Place them on a wide windowsill, or a small table near the light. These are the fruits of the Moon Goddess, now we can recreate that lovely ceremony.

Put a white candle in a small bowl of water and stand it beside the flowers. Light the candle, see the reflection of the flame in the water and think of the beauty and purity of that festival. The women in their white robes, faces shining in the firelight as they work to draw back the light.

Now close your eyes. There is silver moonlight shining in the room— and the sound of the sea. Match your breathing with the steady music of the waves. As you breathe, draw in the scent of the flowers and visualize another light slowly rising from the water, the warmth of ancestral wisdom. It grows in intensity until it meets the moonlight and the two fuse, bathing the room in lovely pastel shades of early spring: palest yellow, silver-green, turquoise, aquamarine, pink, lilac. . .

Hold these colours in your mind's eye as you inhale the scent of the flowers.

Keep breathing deeply and eventually open your eyes.

I carry Earth's wisdom within me.

PISCES FULL MOON:
CLEANSING MOON

> The three months of Spring are called the period of the beginning. . .the breaths of Heaven and Earth are prepared to give birth, thus everything is developing and flourishing. . .Those who disobey the laws of Spring will be punished with an injury of the liver. *Nei Ching*

We need to cleanse our systems and what better spring cleaner could we have than Lemon, favourite ingredient of every washing up liquid.

LEMON *(Citrus limon)**

The lemon brings the summer sun and has an affinity for the liver: just smelling it will produce the sour taste that the liver needs. A slice of lemon in spring water in the morning will help the liver's function.

Its perfume has a sharp, laser-like effect on the senses, banishing lethargy, and its squeaky-clean freshness cuts through confusion. We need this now to focus all that incoming Arian energy. Lemon diffused in a room not only deals with germs efficiently, but also clears the head. Its direct action on the brain lifts depression and brings us all out of hibernation. It will purge you of any dross that is preventing your progress and its colour is that of the intellect, so use it to sharpen yours.

I do not recommend you meditate with Lemon. Use it when you see the first rays of spring sunshine, and if you really want the freedom and energy to go, blend it with Black Pepper.

* Essence of Lemon can be photosensitive and will sometimes irritate a sensitive skin.

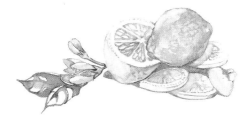

THE EAST WIND
Young and beautiful was Wabun;
He it was who brought the morning,
He it was whose silver arrows
Chased the dark o'er hill and valley;
He it was whose cheeks were painted
With the brightest streaks of crimson,
And whose voice awoke the village,
Called the deer, and called the hunter.

H.W. Longfellow, 'The Four Winds',
The Song of Hiawatha, 1854

To the Indians of the Great Lakes, Wabun brought the fertile energy of Spring. Now, in this season of youth and illumination, his bright colours appear, heralded by the rich maroons, brick reds and yellows of the Wallflower (*Cheiranthus cheiri*). From March until May this 'forty-day flower' speaks to us of Earth's abundant energy. Decked out in Wabun's clothes, these cheerful velvet blooms leave a rich, heady scent lingering in the air. As yet there is no natural essence available, but a clump of these delightful flowers in the garden will more than compensate. With hints of Narcissus, Rose and Jasmine, the fragrance holds the promise of summer, but keeps us yearning, like the poet said, to 'have it ever spring'.

*A*RIES NEW MOON:
SPRING WINDS MOON

This new moon is influenced by the cosmic activity of the Equinox and is often a time of high winds and unsettled weather. The waxing Aries moon brings an upsurge of growth and, like the Ram of the Zodiac turning over new soil with his horns, there is a feeling of discovery, of developing a new relationship with the environment. It may be the same one you inhabited last year, but both of you have entered a new cycle. The instinctive response is heightened at this time.

BLACK PEPPER *(Piper nigrum)*
Full of resilience and vigour, this courageous oil is one for the moment. Like Clove, this is another stalwart of the spice trade and has similar associations with wealth and security. Black pepper, however, is intent on victory. With a fragrance that is hot, dry and sweetly penetrating, it represents wilful energy. It keeps away negativity, and protects you on

short journeys or transactions. It is good for this rapidly moving time of year.

For those who are afraid to be ruthless when necessary, Black Pepper turns anger into a positive force. It puts thoughts into action and encourages openness over needs and wants. Use it occasionally to activate rather than meditate; this way it will give you a sense of presence and help you to get to the point. Use it sparingly and it will not tire your senses; use it indiscriminately and, like the energy of Mars, its ruler, it will overpower you and make you lose your head.

SPRING EQUINOX: MARCH 21ST: EQUAL DAY AND NIGHT

The Vernal Equinox is Nature's balancing act when the magnetic forces of light and dark are locked together. As light overcomes darkness, everything starts to vibrate at a faster rate, the adrenalin flows, and the masculine force rises with renewed vigour. Body warmth and fluid, conserved during the winter, starts to shift once more, but without proper direction it may stagnate, giving rise to spring ailments. Something is needed to help it along.

COMMON THYME *(Thymus vulgaris* – and other species)

> It is a strengthener of the lungs; a good remedy for the
> chin-cough in children. It purges the body of phlegm,
> and is an excellent remedy for the shortness of breath.
>
> Nicholas Culpeper, *The English Physician*, 1653

Thyme directs the energy outwards, radiating heat from the centre towards an outgoing, joyful attitude to life. Now is the time for sharing and expressing all that creativity you have been harbouring during the winter.

If Black Pepper is the warrior, Thyme is the tireless Red Cross worker. Associated with chivalry and bravery, it has known field hospitals from the Crusades to the Crimea. This powerful antiseptic was used to fight Yellow Fever and scrub hospital floors up to the Great War.

For such an extrovert, however, Thyme displays great humility, growing on the poorest soil and giving up its essence willingly. Rich and poor have strewn it across their floors for centuries. It has had a special relationship with children, and is very useful for dealing with any inward looking, introverted behaviour. The herb was used to line the mattresses of cradles and prevent nightmares. Stimulating, yet balancing, it is not a scent to promote sleep as such, but one to banish the bogey man from under the bed!

Just one whiff of its invigorating scent makes you feel healthy. Use it to banish petty fears, dark thoughts and winter woes.

Thyme can transmute itself through a very wide range of scents and properties, depending on where it is grown. There are those with a red pungency and those that are gentle and extremely refined. Be guided by your therapist or supplier. Some Thymes can irritate the skin.

MEDITATION: THYME

This is a nice spring meditation to do beside an open fire.

Sit quietly with a few drops of Thyme in a burner and take a healthy, honest look at your life. What is motivating you at present? What direction are you going in? Examine the positive and negative influences, the ones that are closest to you, in your home or your working environment. Are you being straightforward about what you want, or are you merely drifting?

Thyme works to bring more basic instincts into harmony with the emotional centre. Breathe deeply and steadily and imbibe the radiating warmth of the fragrance. Place your hands together just below the navel.

Breathe in:	Expand your tummy and draw its warmth inside.
Breathe in	
and out gently:	Visualize a warm red circulating.
Breathe out:	Send its positive influence spiralling outwards.

(Do this two or three times with the red, and then just let it go, as too much can be overpowering.)

Let's get on with it!

ARIES FULL MOON:
EARLY RAINS MOON

GERANIUM (*Pelargonium graveolens cultivar* – and other species)

> ... the April grove, thick with the primrose ... in its
> green dress with true abundance, filled with joy ... the
> bright water, the limpid water, a place of fair wellbeing, a
> place to sleep, a place to learn whole tunes of melody.
>
> Edmund Price, Archdeacon of Merioneth, *The Mansion in the Wood*

There is always one day in April when suddenly
everything, everywhere is covered in green – and it is
raining. Clouds of early perfumes are released into
the air and, for me, the scent of Geranium comes to
mind. Like a soft, refreshing shower, here is the
green balancer, the one which meets the other six
colours half way in the spectrum. Perhaps that is why we
see so much of it in nature.

The essence we use comes from the leaf of a plant that
originates from southern Africa. This calm, refreshing oil
is a great treasure. The action of a balancer is always
difficult to define because it creates harmony
wherever it goes. Its fragrance can vary slightly, but is

a lovely light 'green' which often has rosy undertones. Geranium brings a sense of space and is a good background fragrance for any room, especially if you want to cleanse the atmosphere of chatter, gossip, or inharmonious vibrations. It is tolerant and can adjust to your needs and, under the influence of Venus, it brings a touch of romance. It is the perfect essence to smooth away the raw turbulence of the March winds and take us towards a gentler time of year.

GERANIUM: MEDITATION
Diffuse a little Geranium into the room.

For a sense of space and relaxation of body and spirit, imagine you are standing on the top of a hill with a wide vista all around. In the sky there is a lovely rainbow.

Visualize a white light surrounding everything which gradually turns to a beautiful pale but radiant green. Allow your whole being to move out into this fresh, green space. Explore it, imagine it filled with clean, sweet air. Fill your lungs and allow it to purify your spirit.

Enjoy it and then gradually let the green dissolve into pink then back into white and return to your original space.

These images of colours dissolving into each other help us to understand the changing shades of our own personalities and lives.

Life needs to discover balance.

$\mathcal{E}$ASTER:

FIRST SUNDAY AFTER THE ARIES FULL MOON

Look upon the rainbow, and praise him that made it;
Very beautiful it is in the brightness thereof.
It compasseth the heaven about with a glorious circle,
And the hands of the most High have bended it.

Edmond Bordeaux Szekely,
'The Heavenly Father, *The Essene Gospel of Peace*

All the colours of the spectrum appear in the magnificent, shimmering arch of a rainbow, through the prism of rain and sunshine. Just for a moment we are allowed this glimpse of Nature's geometry – and then it fades. A rainbow is like a perfume, we can never really possess it, it shows us the illusions of our material world.

SWEET VIOLET (*Viola odorata*)

Like the rainbow the natural scent of Violet fades the moment it touches your consciousness. Were you dreaming or did it really happen? An essence from the petals is rare. Attempts have been made to copy its angelic quality, all have failed, but the cool purple of this modest little healer is welcome now, hidden away in damp shady places, often protected by the pale yellow primrose. We must search for them both if we are to appreciate their fragrances.

Music, when soft voices die,
Vibrates in the memory –
Odours, when sweet violets sicken,
Live within the sense they quicken.

Percy Bysshe Shelley, 19th Century

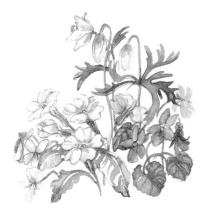

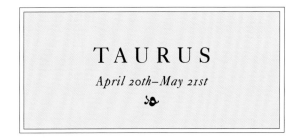

TAURUS

April 20th–May 21st

The Great Spirit is our Father, but the Earth is our Mother. She nourishes us; that which we put into the ground she returns to us, and healing plants she gives us likewise. If we are wounded, we go to our Mother and seek to lay the wounded part against her, to be healed. Animals too, do thus, they lay their wounds to the earth.

Big Thunder, a Native American of the Wabanakis Nation, 1900

TAURUS NEW MOON:
FERTILE MOON

Taurus is the most solid Earth sign of the zodiac, representing the moist fertility of the soil. It brings with it the harmony and tranquillity of its ruler, Venus, allowing us to balance Earth's energy with our own.

VETIVER (*Vetiveria zizanoides/Andropogon muricatus*)

Vetiver comes from a solid root and from a family of plants that has produced some of our most sacred food: wheat, barley, oats, corn, rice, millet, are all relatives. In most mythologies the root is symbolically set in the south, the moist, warm place of feeling and instinct. The tropics of the southern hemisphere are Vetiver's home.

Its smell reminds me of the rich, black earth of old cottage gardens and it is the same dark colour. Immediately strengthening and grounding, but not at all cloying, it always leaves me feeling very clear headed. It strengthens the tissues as it strengthens the will and is used a lot to treat exhaustion. The heat of its native environment gives it an aphrodisiac quality and it has been prized as a perfume in the East for centuries. Sanskrit texts refer to it as an unguent used for anointing brides.

Vetiver touches the primeval in us and shows us the value of earthly instincts. In an urban environment, however, these can often move into the realm of fantasy and need a more realistic base. If you live too much in your head, its simple action is to bring you back to earth. If you sit all day long, it will remind you of the division you have created between mind and body. For all of us it will develop a sense of responsibility, both to ourselves and to the environment.

VETIVER: MEDITATION

To lighten its effect, Vetiver blends well with Lavender or Lemon, or other members of its own family that are coming later in the year. On its own it is effective simply inhaled on a smelling tab just in front of you.

Settle down, face the South, and think of the Earth. Visualize your own roots penetrating deep into the ground and surround yourself with a rich, brown aura. Think of your animals and plants and include them in this meditation. Then think about the essences from an ecological point of view. The plants have to be cared for, harvested and distilled. Many travel long distances to reach us and are handled by people whose cultural and environmental backgrounds are different from our own. We can enjoy the experience of perfume, but must never forget that we are all part of a balance that becomes ever more fragile.

Inhale Vetiver and walk barefoot upon the sacred Earth. Touch her and receive her blessings.

The Earth is our mother, we must care for her.

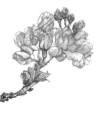

TAURUS FULL MOON: FULL BLOSSOMS MOON

Thou perceivest the Flowers put forth their precious Odours, and none can tell how from so small a centre comes such sweets. . .

William Blake, *Thou Hearest the Nightingale*, 18th Century

As Venus rises higher in the sky, the scent of summer brings an innocent romance to the air.

LINDEN BLOSSOM *(Tilia vulgaris)*

Linden Blossom's thick, gold-brown essence can be solid in the bottle and, like a young heart, often needs warmth if we are to appreciate it. Although beautiful, it is not an erotic fragrance: Linden's is the quality of the early, unbruised blossoms. It touches that innocent spark of first love that flowers briefly before it withers in the gaze of social conditioning. The faintest of memories, the scent of Linden can kiss it alive again, if we let it.

The essence comes from the flower of the Lime Tree. It has a citrus quality which is clean and smooth, but intensely sweet without the cutting edge of Lemon. An emotional cleanser it will clear unwanted or unclean feelings and bring a sense of ease. It soothes nerves, aids sweet sleep and encourages self-confidence, especially in young people. It will put you in touch with your sensuality, but in an innocent, rather than a provocative way.

Use only a tiny amount, and if you find its fragrance heavy, blend with Lemon, or with Lavender which will love its cleanliness.

LINDEN BLOSSOM: MEDITATION

Best done in the morning.

As a child I understood how to give. . .Any pretty pebble was valuable to me then; every growing tree an object of reverence. . .I have forgotten this grace since I became civilized.

Ohiyesa, *The Soul of the Indian*

Linden allows you to become a child again. For this meditation, if you can, visualize pink and blue, the colours of childhood. Put a drop of Linden on a smelling strip and inhale it. Sit comfortably, place one hand in the small of your back and the other below the naval, the fertile energy centre.

Breathe in:	Wrap yourself in the colours as though inside a warm blanket.
Breathe in and out gently:	Think about the vulnerability of a young soul, of your own children or your own childhood. What happened when you got caught doing something naughty? How do you feel when you chastise your own children?
Breathe out:	Allow the blanket to absorb any feelings of shame or guilt that accompany these thoughts.

I acknowledge my Inner Child.

*B*ELTANE:

MAY FESTIVAL

> Merry, it is a momentous thing that the faultless month
> of May is coming, with its heart set on conquering every
> green glen, all hot to assert its rank.
>
> Dafydd ap Gwilym, 'May and January', 14th Century

The Celts greeted this 'time of brightness' with great enthusiasm and everyone mingled at fetes and fairs. May Day was a major fire festival – a real acknowledgement of the sun's power alongside that of the moon.

Now the goddess reappeared as an enchantress to meet her youthful sun god whose home was the universe. Moving towards the more frivolous sign of Gemini, soon came the faerie revellers, with frolics and jokes, jesters and fools, and wonderful dancing colours: saffron, chrome yellow and moss green mingling with the pink and blue of early summer flowers.

For us, this is still a bewitching, vivacious time of colourful flamboyance and liberating energy. Now every young man can be a god and every girl Queen of the May. All Nature is in a process of exchange and communication, giving out its message in perfect harmony.

Natural harmonies are reflected in the way we compose a perfume. The art of blending has been handed down from remote times and one method is to assign each scent to a 'note' on the musical scale – how beautiful!

> The most subtle of all medicines,
> The most potent spell of magic,
> Dangerous more than war or hunting;
> Thus the Love-Song was recorded,
> Symbol and interpretation.
>
> H.W. Longfellow, *The Song of Hiawatha*, 1854

Since the middle ages, romantic music in many cultures has been played on the guitar, an instrument capable of producing a variety of powerfully emotional responses.

Such music is often played in the key of G and on the scale of one famous French perfumer,[*] middle G is given to Orange Blossom, or Neroli. Its essence is the fine pale gold that corresponds to the spiritual colour of the Solar Plexus, the central, emotional centre of the body.

NEROLI (*Citrus aurantium bigaradia*)

Full of youthful loveliness, this delicate white, exquisitely-scented flower is a favourite for bridal bouquets. Its name is taken from a 16th-century duchess and the best essence is expensive, but then so are weddings.

If one were to compare this rich, enticingly heady scent to music, Neroli must surely be a slow waltz, the last waltz, the one before the seduction. In aromatherapy-lore it is tipped as an aphrodisiac with the

[*] Piesse's Scale

55

key quality of allaying any doubts or fears the bride may have concerning her wedding night.

I think this is part of its allure: like a love song, Neroli walks a fine line between innocence and awareness. The petals themselves are delicate tissues clinging to a narrow stem. Brush them carelessly and they fall like snowflakes. This flower reflects the fleeting magic of the wedding night—and so does the scent. At first it has a refreshingly sweet beauty, but let it linger and it starts to cloy. If you are inhaling a cheap variety it could invoke blousey boudoirs instead of chaste marriage beds.

Its reputation for regulating the heart rhythm makes it especially good for anyone who is unable to relax and come to terms with their sexuality. It is more worldly-wise than Linden, but its effect is very comforting. In times of shock or deep anxiety, a tiny amount can be a mild tranquillizer, bringing a sweet relief from deeply-lodged psychological fears. It can be of great value in increasing spirituality and realizing a higher level in a relationship. Be sparing, however, with this song without words, we are no longer in the realms of innocence.

NEROLI: MEDITATION

This exercise is a good one to do before weddings, or any romantic, social event. It is also good after a shock, or any experience which has left your nerves fluttering.

If you find it overpowering to begin with, try blending Neroli with Lavender, Geranium or Lemon.

Sit quietly and listen to the rhythm of your heartbeat. Breathe deeply and place your hands over your navel and make slow, clockwise, circular movements around it. Visualize a pale gold light around you.

If you are in a real state of shock, visualize an orange glow and let it gently dissolve into pink. Orange is sometimes used to treat shock, but needs care.

Inhale the fragrance and let it settle into your soul.

Relax.

I am a quiet reservoir of strength.

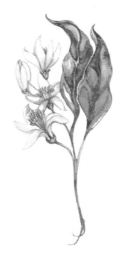

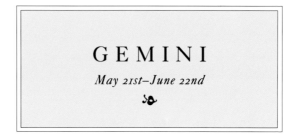

GEMINI

May 21st–June 22nd

. . . summer is on its throne, playing its string-music; the willow, whose harp hung silent when it was withered in winter, now gives forth its melody – Hush! Listen! The world is alive.   Thomas Telynog Evans, 'Winter and Summer'

*G*EMINI NEW MOON:
MOON OF LIGHT AND BEAUTY

This moon takes us towards the Summer Solstice. The sun's influence is strong and a sense of light and space prevails, but this is still a time of great sensitivity and alertness, one of preparation for a greater maturity.

A stone that hath been taken out of the body of a man, being wrapped in camomile, will in time dissolve, and in a little time too.   Nicholas Culpeper, *The English Physician*, 1653

CHAMOMILE (*Chamaemelum nobile*)

The Egyptians dedicated Chamomile to the Sun and she is certainly in love with him for she keeps her face turned towards him always. Garlands of this feminine little flower were found around Tutankhamun's neck, and Chamomile motifs decorated his sandals. What does this tell us? That she was merely walked on by the Pharaoh, as others have walked on her scented lawns for centuries, or did the boy-king really need her gentle, compassionate nature?

Her green aromatic leaves and classic daisy-like face balance mental clarity with purity, but Chamomile hides a deeper secret within. From her the alchemy of distillation extracts a lovely blue substance called azulene with supremely soothing, anti-inflammatory properties.

Her fruity, apple-like fragrance touches vulnerability at a very deep level, finding hidden virtues and drawing out healing energy. All our suffering leads ultimately to a greater understanding of others. Chamomile works on this level, producing a feeling of well-being and security, like a blue blanket of peace. As the essence is reputed to dissolve stones, so the fragrance will soften harsh, self-centred attitudes, the kind we use to drive ourselves as well as others.

It is a fragrance for letting go – gently, without rejecting, loosening the grip of old habits and ideas. It helps if you are being drained of energy, especially by your nearest and dearest and eases the pain of parting, particularly that of mothers and daughters over marriage or leaving home. Soothing and mollifying, helping the flow of energy from the emotional to the heart centre at this still volatile time of year, it can be used whenever its effects are needed.

CHAMOMILE: MEDITATION
Best done in the evening.

I think Chamomile has the ability to draw out suppressed fears and release gentle, feminine wisdom.

There was a time when a woman's menstrual cycle was acknowledged ritualistically. In some societies this was out of respect for a heightened sense of awareness, in others she was just untouchable. Either way, she was set apart at this time. Powerful influences can linger, some say, in the ancestral memory. As that time of the month approaches, archetypal fears can grow as the subconscious prepares the body for an event which these days does not happen. The energy has to go somewhere. Often it manifests simply as a slight change in temperature or awareness, but for those who suffer severely from Premenstrual Syndrome (PMS) it can be strong enough to cause serious disruptions within the family.

The scent of Chamomile is a useful aid when this kind of emotion is welling up. Its nature is so very gentle, use it whenever you are over-stressed and feel you cannot cope. It can bring you back from the edge.

Sit in a warm, dimly-lit room and do the same exercise as for Neroli, but this time visualizing a lovely peaceful blue filling the air, breathe it in and let it permeate your whole being.

And relax.

I trust my feminine energy.

GEMINI FULL MOON:
MOON OF GRACIOUS WISDOM

> The three months of summer are called the period of luxurious growth. The breaths of Heaven and Earth intermingle and are beneficial. Everything is in bloom and begins to bear fruit. . .The pulse is that of the Heart.
>
> *Nei Ching*

This moon, the last full moon before the Summer Solstice, has a special significance, marking the movement of energy to the domain of the heart in both man and nature. Occasionally in the lunar cycle some say that this moon draws the others together by an unseen thread. It represents a period of intense feeling and creativity. A very appropriate fragrance for this time of year is Sandalwood, since this essence has a similar effect on our own energy centres.

SANDALWOOD *(Santalum album)*

This is the scent of the ancient East. Here is an aphrodisiac, but one endowed with spiritual attributes. In Sanskrit it is *chandana* and the Japanese called it *sendan*, bringer of joy.

The wood itself is extremely fragrant – giving off a wonderfully warm, honey-like scent that wraps itself around the senses. Many temples were built from it. The essence comes from the roots and the heartwood, the very heart of the tree, and cannot be obtained until the tree has reached maturity and is felled.[*]

Physically its action is to soothe and lubricate, which is probably the key to its aphrodisiac reputation. It will allow for a greater sexuality, but also enables the senses to move into a higher level of spiritual awareness. Its great value is that it lets us use it for either purpose. Its age-old wisdom has a measuring action, enabling us to savour every moment, and its effect on the psyche is very deep, long-lasting, and of

[*] Technically dead wood, the heartwood is the inner skeleton of the tree and to obtain it, the tree has to be felled. Controls and assurances have been made by the Indian government and aromatherapy constitutes a mere fraction of the entire market. Nevertheless, the use of such essences creates an awareness of the fragile balance that now exists on this planet. (See also Rosewood and Cedarwood.)

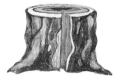

an intimate nature. It encourages an atmosphere of acceptance and openness, but its depth and maturity lessen the anxiety that sometimes accompanies this state. If you live on your nerves, Sandalwood is for you. If you are a placid type you may need to modify your use. If you feel ready to move to a higher level, use Sandalwood regularly in meditation. It will be of great value in unblocking any over-analytical tendencies that get in the way of spiritual development.

Sandalwood is a supremely sustaining oil, nourishment for the soul. Use it to tap into your ancestral memory and release stored wisdom.

SANDALWOOD: MEDITATION

Sandalwood can help us to find the teacher within: the one who understands the pull of earthly desires, but knows the need to find one's own philosophy in life. It is an excellent fragrance for slowing down and stopping a chattering brain.

A good time to do this exercise is if you have a clear evening in front of you when you might decide to do some reading or listen to music.

Put some Sandalwood in a burner. Light a candle and face the East.

Sit quietly and breathe gently as you have done in earlier exercises. Place your hands over your diaphragm.

Visualize a lovely maroon colour rising out of the earth.

Breathe in:	Take the fragrance down to meet it.
Breathe in and out gently:	Be aware of your hands and allow the colour to circulate around the centre.

Now allow the fragrance to attract energy from above in a clear white light which travels down to meet it.

Breathe out: The mingling colours create a soft pink,
                     let your hands go and relax into it.

Do this two or three times and then relax, enjoy the fragrance and let the energy flow by itself.

I can be my own teacher.

SUMMER SOLSTICE JUNE 21ST – LONGEST DAY

> Greeting to you, sun of the seasons, as you travel the skies on high, with your strong steps on the wing of the heights; you are the happy mother of the stars.
>
> Traditional Scottish folk prayer

At last we have reached the time of complete triumph of Light over Darkness – the longest day. At Midsummer the sun has reached its zenith in the sky and the goddess is in complete harmony with Mother Earth. Her natural, lilting harmonies caught the Celtic soul and were celebrated in their poems and songs. Musicians and bards were respected members of the community and travelled among the people carrying the news along with messages of love and guidance.

This tradition was picked up in the middle ages by the Troubadours who, with new philosophies, harmonies and instruments from the East, tried through their songs to revive a spirit of femininity. They are said to have come out of Languedoc, southern France, where the abundance of aromatic herbs and flowers gave rise to the early European perfume industry.

Often shown in paintings with minstrels, lutes and ladies, their emblem of love became the Rose.

R O S E *(Rosa damascena; Rosa centifolia* – and other species)
The most balanced of perfumes, a symphony in itself. As yet unrivalled by commercial imitation, Rose contains many different chemicals so perfectly balanced and in tune with each other that the overall sensation is that of a single scent. Chemists simply cannot reproduce it.

Rose works through the heart to purify and uplift all the other energy centres and from this perfectly-balanced flower we can learn a variety of abilities to keep us properly flowing with life. Midsummer is the time when the Rose reigns supreme as Queen of flowers and its satisfying fragrance is the ideal Guide for a meditation on this day.

It is like a greeting from Heaven. . .unbearably sweet.

Richard Strauss, *Der Rosenkavalier*

Rose represents the force of Heaven on Earth. With its flower in the light and its powerful rootstock anchored firmly in the soil, it shows that earthly desires nourish a greater wisdom – symbolized in the fruit of the rose hips which appear after the flower has withered.

The leaves and petals themselves are arranged in a spiral fashion, receiving the maximum light and energy from the sun. The five heart-shaped petals of the original wild rose were said to correspond to the five-pointed star, symbol of the Microcosm – Man. This may have been the inspiration behind the beautiful rose windows in cathedrals.

To the Arabs, Rose represented the highest spiritual achievement of any flower and they are credited with producing its first essential oil, Attar of Roses. It came from the Damask Rose, or Rose of Damascus which, even now, produces its best essence when grown in that part of the world. Its colour pink is the powerful red of Mars transmuted to a higher spiritual level and it is sometimes given middle C on the musical scale. Venus gives Rose its reputation as the flower of Love and makes it a perfume for the Heart, but not for the faint hearted! This love expresses the courage and compassion to draw out grief and suffering. It can temper the masculine force with a femininity that has the power to heal and nurture on every level.

O, how much more doth beauty beauteous seem
By that sweet ornament which truth doth give!
The Rose looks fair, but fairer we it deem
For that sweet odour which doth in it live.

William Shakespeare, Sonnet 54

ROSE: MEDITATION

Take a deep pink Rose.

Float some petals in a bowl of water and place it near an open window in the setting sun. Add two drops of essence of Rose.

Let the fragrance fill the room. Light a candle, preferably a pink one. Turn off the light, sit down and close your eyes. Relax your whole body.

Breathe softly and evenly for a while. Inhale the fragrance of Rose mingling with the scents of summer.

Breathe in:	Visualize your body filled with a clear white light.
Breathe in and out gently:	Watch the white light turn to a soft pink that envelops you.
	Feel that generous pink light absorbing negativity and grief and transforming them into the nourishment of the Rose which feeds your soul.
	Absorb that compassionate wisdom as it penetrates and revitalizes every cell.
Breathe out:	Think of the qualities the Rose symbolizes.

I am Whole again, joyous in life and love.

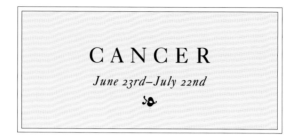

CANCER

June 23rd–July 22nd

This is the only sign of the zodiac under the rulership of the Moon, bringing a sense of beauty and serenity.

CANCER NEW MOON:
MOON OF DELIGHT

This New Moon often falls around the time of the Solstice and if it does it will be especially powerful. But wherever it comes, the next fragrance will enhance the deep, purifying action of Rose.

BERGAMOT (*Citrus bergamia*)[*]
(Do not confuse with the herb *Monarda didyma*, also called Bergamot.)

This bitter fruit produces an essence that is beautiful, refreshing and sweetly citrus with a hint of pear. Legend has it that it is a cross

---

[*] Of all the citrus oils, if applied to the skin, Bergamot has the greatest potential for photosensitivity.

between a pear and a citrus. This is not authenticated, but is easy to believe when one smells it.

A lovely lighthearted green it is, like geranium, a natural balancer which can touch many levels of our psyche.

It is infused with the light and sun of southern Italy, so use it later in the year when our own light is dwindling, your instinct will respond to its sunny friendliness. It is uplifting, but sharpening rather than stimulating, leaving one feeling very 'present'. The supreme room fragrancer, alone or in a blend, it will infuse your life with joy.

Bergamot opens your heart to receive the pure love of the Rose.

BERGAMOT: MEDITATION

I do not recommend you meditate with Bergamot, but it enhances the brain's receptivity to light, so whenever you want to achieve a lighthearted freedom, inhale it to let the sunshine in. It can bring a lovely feeling of weightlessness on hot, oppressive days, so for those people who spend all day in offices, it is excellent in a diffuser to keep the atmosphere cool. It can keep the brain alert, but is not as stimulating as some other fragrances. Some say they wake up, but others say they sleep well after using it.

I feel free.

CANCER FULL MOON:
RADIANCE MOON

Hanging high above the pale gold of the ripening corn, the Full Moon in Cancer is a Lovers' Moon. The mature warmth of summer encourages deeper relationships, especially in the evening when the air is laden with the intoxicating scent of Woodbine, or Honeysuckle.

Honeysuckle's nectar is difficult for bees to reach, so it attracts night flying insects. Sadly, as yet, the essence is rarely available. Imitations fail to capture it, but usually involve blends including other exotics such as Rose, Neroli – and its arch rival, Jasmine.

JASMINE (*Jasminum officinale*)

> Jessamine is a warm, cordial plant, governed by Jupiter
> in the sign of Cancer. . .The oil made by infusion of the
> flowers, is used for perfumes. It disperses crude
> humours. . .   Nicholas Culpeper, *The English Physician*, 1653

With Neroli we enhanced the sensual, with Rose the unconditional, and now we are ready to harmonize the two, as Jasmine completes the love trilogy.

Jasmine's cool, waxy flowers open to the sultry night air and must be

picked before dawn to obtain the fragrance at its
peak. They produce an essence infused with the
sun's glory and the moon's magnetism. Called
'Jessamine' in the West and 'Yasmin' in the East, a drop
of Jasmine in the hand is like a jewel, the gift of a magician
with the ability to transform. This charismatic scent has been a
favourite of sultans and emperors for centuries. Embracing the
rich and beautiful, it dissolves the superfluous and trivial, to smell
it is an ennobling experience.

A guru among oils, given time, it will reveal the truth that hides
behind illusion. Like Sandalwood, it is no stranger to temptation,
but in contrast to Sandalwood's placid nature, Jasmine has a
passionate magnetism whose real and ultimate aim is to burn off base
desire with the fire of eternal love. If you are a realist seeking the
path of higher spiritual endeavour, this is the essence for you.

Diminishing apathy, fear and timidity, this powerful aphrodisiac
works on a mundane level too. Not yet ready for Nirvana? Never mind,
it will help you to deal with Victorian attitudes still lurking behind our
20th-century facade. A master in the art of seduction, as it sets the
scene for romance Jasmine lifts the veil off pretence. Use it during a
waxing moon for success in love and a waning moon to discover
infidelity.

Natural essence of Jasmine is extremely expensive and many tawdry
imitations exist. Take care. Perhaps more than any other oil, true
Jasmine should be handled with the utmost respect. Even a guru is

open to corruption and the greater the wisdom, the harder the fall.
Its majesty overwhelms me, 'I dare write no more of it'.

> My pensive Sara! thy soft cheek reclined
> Thus on mine arm, most soothing sweet it is
> To sit beside our cot, our cot o'ergrown
> With white-flowered Jasmin, and the broad-leaved Myrtle,
> And watch the clouds that late were rich with light. . .
>
> Samuel Taylor Coleridge, 'The Eolian Harp', 19th Century

JASMINE: MEDITATION

For an evening meditation, sit by an open window and look at the beautiful Cancer moon. Invite it into the room.

Put a drop of Jasmine on a smelling strip, or in a burner. Light a candle.

The essence itself is a deep, gold-brown, giving an indication of its ability to draw on more basic energy when necessary. It has such a powerful fragrance that one should not try to work hard whilst inhaling it. A colour I find easy to visualize is a very pale gold and sometimes purple.

Simply breathe gently and slowly and surround yourself with coloured light. As you breathe in allow it to penetrate, feel its rich energy. Breathe out and allow its warmth to remain. Think of the things you would most like to achieve.

By virtue of its cost, if nothing else, Jasmine should be reserved for very special occasions. If you want to achieve something important, imbibe its noble qualities and ask it to carry you through. You can also offer a drop to someone else in honour of a noble cause, I have a friend who always gives some on a handkerchief at Christenings. Or, once in a while, invite your lover to dinner and diffuse a couple of drops into the room – see what happens.

Believe in your dreams.

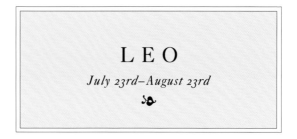

LEO

July 23rd–August 23rd

Traditionally, as the grain ripened, this was always a time of great optimism and confidence, of settling old scores and making new relationships.

*L*EO NEW MOON: SWEET GRAIN –
PREPARATION FOR HARVEST

As reapers sharpened scythes and sickles, corn gods were erected in the fields, soon to be symbolically cut down. In Greek legend this was the busiest time for the goddess, Demeter, and her lovely daughter, Persephone, who joined her from the Underworld. While lonely husband Pluto languished underground, who can blame him for dallying with a practical, though rather pretty little nymph called Menthe? When Persephone found out she was so sick with jealousy, she turned Menthe into a herb.

With his nymph rooted, Pluto's outward ardour cooled, but Menthe kept it warm inside. This is the action of Peppermint.

PEPPERMINT *(Mentha piperita)*

Anyone coming off the hayfield with sunstroke would benefit from Peppermint's cooling properties. In the sultry temperatures of late summer, when body energy is still dispersed towards the surface, Peppermint cools the skin but maintains the inner warmth needed for good digestion. Its light, slightly moisturizing action is cleansing and focussing, clearing heads and refreshing tired minds, but the initial ice-cool effect can be very stimulating and only a tiny amount is needed. It is best avoided at night.

All the mints make wonderful garden plants and their lovely serrated leaves retain their scent for a long time. Dry them and put them in jars around the house to keep the atmosphere clean and bright.

Do not meditate with this oil, simply inhale it to clear your brain, or blend with Lavender, an excellent companion on hot summer days.

LUGNASADH: THE BEGINNING OF HARVEST: 31ST JULY

This was the longest festival, for the harvest lasted from now until the Autumn Equinox. It was dedicated to the Celtic hero Lugh, who has been strongly identified with the god Mercury.

LAVENDER (*Lavandula angustifolia/officinalis*)

> Applied to the temples or nostrils, it reduces the
> tremblings and passions of the heart and faintings and
> swoonings.   Nicholas Culpeper, *The English Physician*, 1653

The scent of Lavender can travel through the senses, touching the
higher spiritual realms or reaching down to basic instincts. All the
masters are in agreement, this plant is ruled by Mercury, whose liquid
energy moves about with ease. It is a truly versatile healer.

Lavender's warmth fortifies the general metabolism, but its cooling
effect on the brain can deal with moodiness, migraines, palpitations or
hysteria. The lovely purplish-blue flowers tell us it is a master healer.
Reach for it whenever extra help is needed. A good quality Lavender
oil is safe for the skin and is often used to soothe cuts and burns.

This well-ordered plant has centuries of clean living behind it. Its
regular, silvery leaf formation tells us it has high ideals and likes to
conform. Its name comes from the Latin *lavare*, to wash, and it was added
to many a Roman bath. Such a practical essence may not have a very
romantic image, but some lavenders can smell quite beautiful, depending
on season and habitat. Since the demand for it is high, so is the
temptation to tamper in order to meet commercial expectations. Beware!

LAVENDER: MEDITATION

This is useful when there is an argument brewing, a feeling of dissatisfaction or a lack of harmony. Sit down with a few drops of Lavender in the burner or on a handkerchief.

Close your eyes, breathe gently and visualize a wide river. In the middle of the river is a beautiful tree covered in mauve flowers. You would love to reach it, but know you cannot cross the water, so you simply sit there admiring it. You become aware of someone in the water, swimming towards you. They are offering you a small branch from the tree. The colour of the blossoms radiates outwards and the fragrance is everywhere. You accept the branch and as you inhale the fragrance your surroundings melt away and are filled with a soft mauve light. Slowly open your eyes.

I gratefully accept Nature's gifts.

*L*EO FULL MOON:
THE HARVEST MOON

All the wild rice has been gathered,
And the maize is ripe and ready;
Let us gather in the harvest,
Let us wrestle with Mondamin,
Strip him of his plumes and tassels,
Of his garments green and yellow!

H.W. Longfellow, 'Blessing the Cornfields',
The Song of Hiawatha, 1854

The ritual cutting down of the Corn God at harvest marks an important division in the lives of many different cultures. Called Mondamin by the Indians of the Great Lakes, he has been identified with the Celtic hero, Lugh, the god Mercury and also Osiris who, it is said, taught the ancient Egyptians how to cultivate grain. This event changed them from a hunter-gatherer society to settled, agricultural people with a degree of control over their environment. The ears of wild grain shatter when they are ripe, releasing their seeds to the wind, whereas those of cultivated grains do not, so they can be stored. The taming of this most independent of plants had a special significance in the development of mankind.

> Then Joseph said unto the people, Behold, I have bought you this day and your land for Pharaoh: lo, here is seed for you, and ye shall sow the lands. Genesis 47:23

Most grains are grasses from the same enormous family as Vetiver. They have spreading, interconnecting root systems which give them a high degree of stability. In some areas such as bushland, grasses replace trees in religious significance. Those from the northern hemisphere have very little colour or perfume.

Further south, however, especially in the tropics, we find some that produce refreshingly beautiful scents such as Lemongrass and Palmarosa.

LEMONGRASS (*Cymbopogon citratus* and *flexuosus*)
This virile grass can be harvested three or four times a year and yields a

stimulating, sometimes slightly aggressive oil. An early-morning essence in every sense of the word, open the bottle and rays of tropical sunshine leap out.

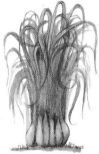

The essence is an opaque yellow-gold and its virility is reflected in its scent. The predominant note is Lemon, but with a denser, more resilient quality. It is a very cheerful pick-me-up with the effect of breezing through the mind. The lovely, lively fragrance helps one to deal easily with unpredictable events of an every day nature. If you have been taken by surprise, involved in any knock-about activities, sports, or simply jostled around on the tube, it will set you up again in no time.

An antiseptic tonic, it makes an excellent room freshener, but especially at this time of year when late summer humidity encourages fungal infections, mosquitoes and flies.

It is not a spiritual plant, but demonstrates the practicality and service of the family it comes from.

PALMAROSA (*Cymbopogon martinii*)

A graceful, feminine grass, Palmarosa bears tiny flowers and loves to float her fragrance like a vesper onto the warm night air. She has a fine, slightly capricious scent: linger with her and she will play little games with your senses. Freshly green and very reminiscent of Geranium, she has shades of other flowers. Was that a hint of rose? Could be, she is a favourite for adulterating that essence. Or was it orange blossom?

Tenderly, she brushes across the mind, this scent is a little posy in itself. Such fragrances are valuable because they test our reactions and provide good exercise for developing an instinctive response. Palmarosa is friendly and loves to be with other essences. A balancer on a slightly more ethereal level than Geranium, she reflects a paler green which tempers richer fragrances. I love her.

LEMONGRASS AND PALMAROSA: MEDITATION
Either of these fragrances is useful diffused into a room in late summer to bring a lighthearted atmosphere. Palmarosa is especially useful in introducing a gentle romance into the air.

They symbolize the spirit of the harvest, one of happiness, singing and dancing. A time of communication, particularly via the throat energy centre. To the Celts this was *cantlos* – 'Song Time' and folk music with flutes and fiddles is often associated with it.

Like the music, these fragrances bring light, air and a lovely expression of emotion, but one that has learnt some control and can therefore afford to sit back and listen to the Pipes of Pan with complete enjoyment.

I do not recommend you meditate with Lemongrass, but with Palmarosa you could use the one given for Geranium, perhaps in the garden, listening to the early evening sounds and replacing the pink with a very pale lilac. As the year moves on, the colours become more translucent – see if you can visualize this.

It is OK to let go.

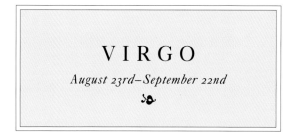

VIRGO

August 23rd–September 22nd

An Earth sign, but ruled by Mercury, Virgo has a soft majesty. She sees the harvest through and brings a gentle prosperity before the onset of Winter.

*V*IRGO NEW MOON:
DANCING WINDS MOON

And the South-Wind o'er the prairie
Wandered warm with sighs of passion,
With the sighs of Shawondasee,
Till the air seemed full of snowflakes,
Full of thistledown the prairie.

H.W. Longfellow, 'The Four Winds',
The Song of Hiawatha, 1854

CARDAMOM *(Elettaria cardamomum)*

As the gentle South Wind blows himself into the arms of wise old Mudjeekewis, from the West, clouds of ripe seeds and pollen float freely on the air.

The delicate seed pods of Cardamom are light as gossamer, the slightest breeze could blow them away. This is a delightful fragrance, but there is no need to buy the essence. I keep a small jar of the seeds in the kitchen and can never resist lifting the lid each time I pass, the perfume quite literally takes my breath away.

The scent of Cardamom is infused with light and warmth from the high mountains of Southern India, which are its natural home. First impression is of a dry, spicy sweetness, but there is another quality that settles round my consciousness in a silken cloud and is difficult to define. Momentarily, whenever I smell it, I leave this place. Where it takes me I cannot say, but I return clear-headed and with a profound sense of simply 'being here'.

One of the 'spices of Caesar', this settling remedy was used by the Arabs as a heart tonic and the Egyptians mixed it with lilies and myrrh to make unguent cones which they placed on their heads. Melting in the heat of the sun, the fragrance spread all over their bodies. Unguent cones were also used by the Hebrews.

> It is like the precious ointment upon the head, that ran down upon the beard, even Aaron's beard: that went down to the skirts of his garments.   Psalms 133:1–2

Wealthy spice merchants were very ruthless, yet they left clear descriptions of the uplifting effects of walking through a spice warehouse. Cardamom must surely have been one of the fragrances to inspire them. Its scent is full of soft voices, flutes and whistles, like the breath of late summer when seed pods fly, carrying their sealed messages into unknown worlds.

CARDAMOM: MEDITATION

I think you have to find your own way with this blithe spirit. It lends itself very well to being sniffed like smelling salts when necessary, but the key phrase is 'in moderation'. Respect it and do not overdo it. If you inhale it late in the evening you might get a wonderfully light and open feeling, but it could prevent sleep.

For me it brings a clear head and a sense of being gently grounded, but with one foot on a golden ladder leading somewhere else. The colours that come to mind are sapphire blue, sometimes with a translucent yellow or pink.

With care it blends beautifully with Jasmine. As yet I have not worked much with this combination, but I have a feeling it could be extremely powerful.

I am open to life's mysteries.

VIRGO FULL MOON:
RIPENING MOON

Season of mists and mellow fruitfulness,
Close bosom-friend of the maturing sun;
Conspiring with him how to load and bless
With fruit and vines that round the thatch-
eves run. . .   John Keats, 'To Autumn', 1819

Fruit picking follows harvest. Ripe fruits are natural fertility symbols and under this beautiful orange moon, with the horn of plenty overflowing, the scent of Patchouli comes to mind.

PATCHOULI *(Pogostemon cablin)*
It lives in the tropics and its large leaves must be fermented before the brown, sticky essence can be obtained. It has a sultry and very enduring perfume, earthy, but musty and smoky, not the clay-like smell of Vetiver. Patchouli keeps very well and actually improves with age.

Within this sweet enveloping perfume one can detect a raw instinct, but this one deepens human relationships as well as environmental ones. Used by people who are getting on in life, its effect can be one of rejuvenation, of reawakening and rediscovering the mystery and excitement of early sexual attraction.

Like autumn leaves falling, Patchouli symbolizes the return to a fertile earth. Feeding and enriching, it allows us to continue life's cycle with renewed energy, stability and the wealth of experience accumulated during the year.

Its effect can be deepened by blending it with Sandalwood or lightened by Palmarosa. A fruitful way to end the summer. Whatever Nature takes from the soil, she returns in greater abundance.

Do not meditate with this essence, simply use it to create a more fruitful atmosphere or when you need to relax.

Autumn Equinox 21st September Equal Night and Day

> The whole land, every dale and glen, weeps its long sorrow after the graceful summer; no tree-top can do more nor weep leaves after that.
>
> Thomas Nicholson, 'An Epigram'

The Autumn Equinox has the strong magnetic pull of spring, but this time light is being overpowered by darkness and there is a greater sense of foreboding. For some time before or after we can experience temperature changes and often spectacular electric storms.

At Imbolg the energy rose gently from the water, but here the two irreconcilable elements confront each other. Fire dancing on water, the purifying force steams and hisses as it burns off the watery surface of the deep. This cracking or splitting of the atmosphere fascinated our ancestors and can still provoke powerful images of abrupt changes in destiny.

Fear of an external unseen force can be very debilitating. Such fears have a mercurial quality, appearing when least expected or desired, sometimes giving rise to deep depression or paranoid behaviour.

CLARY SAGE (*Salvia sclarea*)

> It is a usual course with many men, when they have got the running of the reins, or women the whites, to run to the bush of Clary, exclaiming – Maid, bring hither the frying-pan, and fetch me some butter quickly. Then they will eat fried Clary just as hogs eat acorns, and this they think will cure their disease, forsooth!
>
> Nicholas Culpeper, *The English Physician*, 1653

Here is an oil that commands respect and cannot be dictated to. Of course, no essence can really. They work holistically and each one is unique in producing the effect that the body needs at that particular time.

Sometimes called 'clear eye', Clary Sage is liquid light. Like Mercury, it is an astral traveller, moving with ease through the emotional spectrum with the ability to open up new vistas of experience. These sometimes come through dreams, bringing a long and deeply relaxing sleep, followed by a release of creativity. For the occasional few, though, it might be a night of unbridled restlessness.

The essence is from the leaves. Respect it, abandon yourself to its influence, it will relax your body wonderfully while it leaves your mind clear and open. Unlocking unseen doors and clearing emotional debris, its resilience allays the anxieties of modern life and evokes higher influences. I have used it effectively to remove 'writer's block' whilst working on this book.

Some are tempted to use Clary in the same way as an hallucinatory drug. This is futile. Its equivocal nature enjoys having fun: misuse it and it will simply tease you. Its appearance says it all. Huge jagged leaves and a tall flowering stem that sits jauntily, often with a sideways droop. Clary is the jester in disguise.

The flowers, though, are the deep mauve of the master healer. Tiny, with half closed mouths, they tell us Clary can keep a secret. Its fragrance is often an acquired taste and is difficult to define since it, too, crosses boundaries. Fresh, slightly bitter-sweet, almost the scent of a freshly cracked hazelnut. Warm, penetrating, yet incisive, it leaves me with a lovely feeling of expansion. Stand alone in a field of Clary Sage and you will never go home. You will not stand for long either, as collectively the fragrance is intoxicating.

CLARY SAGE: MEDITATION

Sometimes we can detect patterns in our own behaviour that we know are blocking creativity, but which we simply cannot shift. If you would like to begin to erode some of these, start very gently by inhaling Clary. This is best done in the evening, shortly before going to bed, no more than once a week.

Once again, put a couple of drops in a burner and light a candle. Blend with Lavender, Orange or Sandalwood to lighten the effect.

Sit with your back straight, but fully relaxed.

Breathe very deeply and regularly and inhale the uplifting fragrance.

Breathe in:	Allow the fragrance in and visualize a current of white energy running down your spine.
Breathe in and out gently:	The current vibrates to a soft, translucent lilac.
Breathe out:	Let that energy release itself and as it goes, send the colour spiralling away from you.
Relax:	Watch the lilac disperse into white and as it does, it sends a lovely shower of rainbow colours all over you. Then it all dissolves into white again.

Do this two or three times and then simply relax and breathe gently and deeply for about five minutes and think very positively about the beautiful things in your life.

I feel secure – I can open any door.

Do not drink or drive after inhaling Clary Sage.

LIBRA

September 23rd–October 24th

♎

LIBRA NEW MOON:
MOON OF CHANGING SEASONS

Sweet thy breath is as the fragrance
Of the wild flowers in the morning,
As their fragrance is at evening,
In the Moon when leaves are falling.

H.W. Longfellow, 'Hiawatha's Wedding Feast',
The Song of Hiawatha, 1854

Autumn can be compared with the twilight of life, the middle years when general activity slows down and a greater wisdom starts to emerge. Its light has a translucent quality with shades of copper and gold, topaz and amethyst, delicate vibrations that reflect the energy of the beautiful, slow-growing Rosewood.

ROSEWOOD (*Aniba rosaeodora*)

> There is another land which it would be no worse to
> seek; the sun sets, I see it – though it is far, we shall
> reach it before night.   Irish, anon, 8th Century

Rosewood comes from the bark of a tree that grows in the Brazilian rain forest, and to obtain the essence the tree must be felled.[*] Its warm, light, syrupy fragrance delights the senses, stroking them gently. I love it. Its perfume is concerned with the finer fabric of the intellect as it seeks perfection. Working on a cerebral level, it encourages new and more creative thought forms if one is open to receive them. It has shown itself to be of particular value to those working in the arts, especially photography and film.

It is a healer of scar tissue, both physical and mental. It will encourage sensuality, but to use it specifically for this purpose will only jar the emotions, for its essential nature is one of amiable spirituality. Rosewood is for seekers, especially those who have become disillusioned and wander from one persuasion to another, aimlessly seeking the right path. It has a lingering enchantment that can turn languishing into longing and longing into realization. It lets us stop, breathe deeply, sigh even. If we are ready we will attract like-minded seekers.

---

[*] Assurances have been made by the Brazilian government – see also Sandalwood.

ROSEWOOD: MEDITATION

In the pursuit of learning, every day something is acquired.

In the pursuit of Tao, every day something is dropped.

Lao Tsu, *Tao Te Ching*

Rosewood offers a station along the road, a stopping-off point to revive one's spirits and offload unnecessary luggage, aspects of life that are no longer necessary. As one climbs higher, the fewer items of baggage the better. This can also be done with Sandalwood or Cedarwood.

Light a candle and put a couple of drops of Rosewood into a burner.

Sit quietly and breathe gently and evenly.

Allow a feeling of slow timelessness to rise up and surround you. Relax into it.

You are walking through a wood, carrying a heavy bag.

You arrive at a clearing where you see a well with a wooden drinking cup beside it. You take some of the clear water, rest awhile, and then you move on. The sun is shining through the canopy of leaves and you feel lighthearted – and light. You realize you have left the bag behind you.

I can move on, there are no restrictions

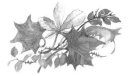

*L*IBRA FULL MOON:
MOON OF TRANQUILLITY

More majestic than the silken canopy
Of the rich merchant,
Is the tent of branches above my head.

Edmond Bordeaux Szekely, 'Trees',
The Essene Gospel of Peace, Book Two

Man has always had a special relationship with trees. They are his link between Earth and Heaven. They support him, breathing in his waste, transforming and transporting it high into the air. Trees stand against the landscape and give it focus. They are timeless, carrying messages from the past and providing us with our most spiritually uplifting essences.

CEDARWOOD (*Cedrus atlantica*)

Now therefore command them that they hew me cedar
trees out of Lebanon.   I Kings 5:6

The cedars for Solomon's temple came from Mount Lebanon where there was a vast forest of them. He was not the first to take them, the Egyptians had been felling them for years. Cedar was prized for its resistance to bugs and fungus, but also for its fragrance. Like

Sandalwood, it released its scent into the atmosphere in temples and other buildings where people gathered to worship.

> Through the rugged oak and the royal cedar,
> The Earthly Mother has sent a message of love
> To the Heavenly father.
>
> Edmond Bordeaux Szekely, from 'Trees',
> *The Essene Gospel of Peace*, Book Two

Once, like the Druids under the oaks in Britain, the people of the Middle East loved these majestic trees and used the forests as temples in their own right, worshipping in the natural fragrance of the open air.

'First Quality Cedar Oil' was one of the sacred embalming oils of the Egyptians and, like Myrrh, was associated with the safe passage of the soul to the next life. Linked with the handsome god Horus, it would bring beauty, dignity and majesty to the soul in its future life.

Our essence comes from the shavings of a close relative, a tall, powerful tree called Atlas Cedarwood. It must not be confused with Virginian Cedarwood (*Juniperus virginiana*) and some other members of the Juniper family which are the cedars referred to in American Indian smudging ceremonies.

The essence itself has a light, liquid gold texture with a fragrance that has the same honey-like quality as Sandalwood, but is not as sweet.

Like the great kings whose souls it entered, it radiates wisdom on a grand scale. The scent of Cedar evokes the sacred geometry of buildings, secret knowledge transferred to the stones of temples and cathedrals. This universal essence is a valuable aid for deep breathing and makes a wonderful room fragrancer to prepare a group of people for meditation and contemplation.

Cedar is a perfume for the brow energy centre and is concerned with higher intuition and communication.

CEDARWOOD: MEDITATION

This is the time of year when we should be building our own temple. An imaginary one that we can retreat to on cold winter nights. Metaphoric temples, huts and mansions appear a lot in Celtic poetry. They are often described with a gemstone in the centre, symbolizing the purity of the soul.

> Its candlesticks are golden, with a candle of great purity, with a gem of precious stone in the very middle of the house. Anon, 12th/13th Century, *Iubhdhan's Fairy House*

Build your temple with Cedar of course. Put a few drops in a burner and light a candle.

Sit down and close your eyes and breathe deeply and evenly.

First put an imaginary circle around you, and fill it with white light: this is the foundation. Now visualize whatever construction you feel comfortable with. It can be a little room, or a bower under the skies with a thatched roof. Whatever it is, it will be a place to go to for healing and learning whenever you need it. Feel your own limitations within its boundaries. Understand that you can expand them as you grow. If there is a problem on your mind when you enter the room, leave it outside and close the door. Give yourself a rest from it just for that period of time. Sit down, fill the room with light and breathe gently for 5 or 10 minutes.

Relax, the problem may be smaller than you think.

See what colour Cedar evokes for you. But you do not always have to do this visualization with Cedar, once you have built the temple you can use it whenever you feel you need it.

I can heal myself.

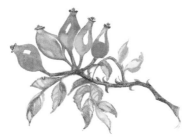

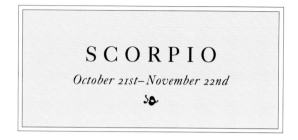

SCORPIO

October 21st–November 22nd

Soul and Spirit should be gathered together in order to make the breath of the Fall tranquil. . .   *Nei Ching*

The ceremonial life of many ancient cultures came alive during the winter months when people gathered to listen to myths and stories passed down by their elders. Taking the form of dramatic performances with music, colourful masks and perfumed incense, these events could make a deep and important connection within the fabric of their lives. Here, behind the shield of fantasy, people were able to relive the events of the year, releasing fears and phobias within the safety of the community.

As these traditions moved into the confines of the temple, they were presided over by priests. In Egypt especially, this practice was transformed into a highly sophisticated healing art. The spirits of our ancestors were sometimes personifications of the shades of emotion that are so familiar today. In their ritualistic way perhaps they faced them more squarely than we do.

SCORPIO NEW MOON:
MOON OF WISE WITHDRAWAL

But when the melancholy fit shall fall
Sudden from heaven like a weeping cloud.

John Keats, 'Ode on Melancholy', 1819

The clocks are going back, you've caught your first cold of the season and you're feeling S.A.D.

S.A.D. – Seasonal Affective Disorder – is a condition attributed in part to the waning light. It can bring on a profound feeling of isolation and hopelessness. People suffering from S.A.D., or any type of depression, often wish they could hibernate. Part of the treatment is to stand in front of a 'daylight lamp'.

'Then glut thy sorrow on a morning rose'. . .Keats was right, and now is the time to bring out many of the sunny essences you have in your collection.

MELISSA (*Melissa officinalis*)

The Arabian physicians have extolled the virtues thereof to the skies. . .it causeth the mind and heart to become merry. . .driveth away all troublesome cares and thoughts out of the mind, arising from melancholy and black choler. . .   Nicholas Culpeper, *The English Physician*, 1653

Traditionally called 'Balme' and sometimes 'heart's delight', Melissa holds its delightful essence in the flowers and pretty heart-shaped leaves. Its compassionate nature is similar to that of Chamomile, but whilst that fragrance penetrates deeply, Melissa's effect is more one of throwing a canopy of light around us. Its essence is pale yellow with a rich, smooth lemon scent that provokes happy, sunny images, helping us to find beauty in our surroundings. Tradition has it that it is best picked on Midsummer's Day.

> . . .the hives of Bees, being rubbed with the leaves of Bawne, causeth the Bees to keep together, and causeth others to come unto them.
>
> John Gerard, *The History of Plants*, 1597

For depression, paranoia, hypochondria, this essence is good. Under its protective screen one experiences a feeling of warmth, like the inside of a hive. Here everything is friendly and the gremlins and nagging voices of doubt are locked out. Use it to line your own imaginary temple and to disperse loneliness, fear and sadness.

The herb has been an ingredient of syrups, elixirs and healing salves for centuries. It is your gentle tonic for any dark, depressing days. It blends well with Lavender, Geranium, Rose and some of the spice oils.

MELISSA: MEDITATION
Melissa is often used to treat allergies and is one of the best remedies

for those who are allergic to life. It can show us the beauty of our immediate surroundings. If you are feeling depressed on a dark winter's day, take it into your imaginary healing room.

Go inside and close the door.

Light a candle and put a drop of Melissa in a burner or on a smelling strip in front of you. If you want to achieve extra balance, blend it with Geranium.

Sit quietly and inhale the fragrance.

Visualize a golden light all around you, filling the room. Outside rain is falling, but the walls absorb all the vibrations. Inside it is warm and green grass grows all around, with daisies, primroses and a clear, running stream.

Breathe gently and evenly, with your hands just beneath your diaphragm and enjoy being there.

After a while, take an extra deep breath in and feel your body tingling with life.

Then, with each out-breath, allow the golden light to become more intense and to start moving outwards, taking the roof with it. You keep on breathing and there is a lovely feeling of expansion. Through the light you can see blue sky. It has stopped raining. You walk outside again and raise your arms.

'Hush! Listen! The world is alive.'

SAMHAIN (HALLOWE'EN):
31ST OCTOBER

There were times in Celtic life when law and order was dismantled to allow the people some respite from daily routines and at Samhain deliberate chaos reigned. Doors banged, animals moved about, neighbours slept in different houses, witches were abroad, things literally went bump in the night.

This was the Celtic New Year, and for one night the spirits of departed loved ones were invited in to sit at the hearth and be fed and cared for. This is reminiscent of our own New Year 'first footing' tradition. When the night was over, the ancestors were taken to the village boundaries and seen off with clattering bells and drums – and the goddess too, now the old hag of Hallowe'en, vanished into the unseen world. Symbolically dying, she went underground where her transformation continued unseen until the magnetic force of spring drew her out as a maiden once again.

This spirit of death and rebirth is honoured through another lovely tree, the Cypress.

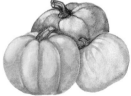

CYPRESS (*Cupressus sempervirens*)

> The wind among the leaves of the cypress
> Maketh a sound like unto a chorus of angels.
>
> Edmond Bordeaux Szekely, from 'Trees',
The Essene Gospel of Peace, Book Two

Cypress has long been associated with the protective aspect of death. This very beautiful tree has a powerful aura with deep blue-green branches which form a dense cone shape, pointing upwards. Immensely strong and resistant, collectively these trees can form a shield and are a favourite windbreak, especially around cemeteries.

The essence comes from the leaves and cones and the fragrance has a slightly sharp masculinity with a woody centre. It has a quality that moves the senses upwards, like the branches of the tree itself. The overall effect is one of sweetness.

> Sweeter than the finest nectar
> Of the honeyed pomegranate
> Is the fragrance of the wind
> In the grove of cypress.
>
> Edmond Bordeaux Szekely, 'The Angel of Air',
The Essene Gospel of Peace, Book Two

The scent of Cypress can ease the flow of emotional tears, especially those of parting. At times of great loss it is of value in developing an understanding that death is merely a continuum from one existence into another. It can help those with loved ones who are close to death, or the dying themselves who may be reluctant to leave this plane, allowing both sides the freedom to let go. If someone has had a near-death experience, Rose or Neroli will ease the initial shock or trauma, but Cypress will deal with the understanding and coming to terms with what has happened.

Cypress can also ease the transitions that are part of life, such as changing one's attitude towards something or someone. For people who tend to take a hard line, it shows a more lenient approach. It also helps to overcome fear of the dark, or the unknown, and of course the fear of death itself.

Death is not always peaceful and Cypress does not deny the agony of any loss or tragedy, but it is concerned with facing the truth, and as such will lift the spirits out of introspection and into the light.

> Let him be just and deal kindly with my people, for the dead are not powerless. Dead – I say? There is no death. Only a change of worlds.
>
> Chief Seattle (on surrendering his land in 1885 –
> the city of Seattle now stands there)

CYPRESS: MEDITATION

Hallowe'en is a good time to think of all the gentle cultures and societies who lost the battle for survival against more aggressive civilizations. Technically dead they may be, but their philosophies and beliefs live on and are being reborn. Now it seems, there is a desperate rush to clutch at the remaining fragments of their wisdom, as if to paper over the cracks in our own culture.

As you inhale the fragrance of Cypress, tune in to whichever one you feel closest to, or think generally if that is easier.

You can also use it at any time to deal with death or transition. Moving house, changing jobs, changing direction: as we saw with Myrrh, life is full of little deaths.

(Whenever I smell Cypress I cannot help but visualize its own deeply penetrating blue-green colour.)

Life is full of little deaths.

EUCALYPTUS (*Eucalyptus globulus* – and other species)

> When people are hurt by the humidity of the Fall,
> they will get a cough in Winter.   *Nei Ching*

I do not recommend this oil for meditation, but the essence from this beautiful evergreen tree is valuable as a room fragrancer, to release natural antibiotics into the atmosphere, especially in winter. The powerful psychological message carried by its scent greatly enhances its physical action.

It blends well with Lemon.

$\mathcal{S}$CORPIO FULL MOON:
MOON OF MODERATION

> . . .people should suppress and conceal their wishes as
> though they had no internal purpose. . .all this is the
> method for the protection of one's storing. *Nei Ching*

To the Celts this was the 'darkest depths' when all that was surplus had
been dispensed with and only the vital elements returned to the earth
for rebirth. Now we should examine our own watery depths and read
the legacy of the old year. Many attitudes and habits will be frozen and
revived next thaw, but a few might be transmuted during the winter
months into something more positive.

  The next essence has long been respected and comes from a family
whose members look so similar that it is often difficult to tell them
apart. With their tall, waving stems and characteristic umbrella-like
heads, plants from the Parsley family have delighted our stomachs
down the ages. Angelica, aniseed, caraway, chervil, coriander, cumin,
dill, fennel, even carrot and parsnip – with such a tempting variety to
stimulate his appetite, one fancies that man has had an easy
relationship with this family. Not so. The plants themselves can smell
unpleasant and potential poisoners such as Hemlock lurk within their
ranks. Nature never lets us take her for granted.

> And Moses said unto them, This is the bread which the
> Lord hath given you to eat. . .And the House of Israel
> called the name thereof Manna: and it was like
> Coriander seed, white; and the taste of it was like wafers
> made with honey.   Exodus 16:15 and 31

CORIANDER (*Coriandrum sativum*)

The seed of Coriander is carried within a hard outer coating of fruit,
combining strength with a sense of economy. The plant has a nauseous
smell, but crush the cream-coloured fruit of Coriander
and you release a delicious scent with a smooth,
silky texture, well rounded but containing many
different shades. Is it like 'wafers made with
honey'? It can add a rich, creamy quality to
other fragrances. A musky undertone with a
faint hint of aniseed, I find it a most intriguing
fragrance.

Coriander is a dependable storehouse of
energy. Similar to Black Pepper, but whilst
Pepper is outgoing, Coriander embodies
conserved, controlled courage, the kind that is in
command and does not dissipate itself with
unnecessary physical or mental activity. It is a
Samurai warrior, bringing a sense of rhythm, even
poetry, to strength. It can turn nervousness into

creative energy and temper irritability.

Coriander is for accepting total responsibility for one's actions and allowing the leader within to emerge. Like all accomplished warriors, this supremely confident fragrance maintains an air of living dangerously. Use it before an important interview, or a meeting with your mother-in-law!

In excessive doses, can be stupefying.

CORIANDER: MEDITATION

> Better stop short than fill to the brim.
> Oversharpen the blade, and the edge will soon blunt.
>
> Lao Tsu, *Tao Te Ching*

This is a lovely description of self-control. That is what Coriander teaches us. It blends well with other essences, a good mixer yet with a total belief in itself. You can add it to Cypress, Clary Sage, Neroli, Sandalwood, Bergamot, Pine, Ginger: it will enhance their action.

When you inhale Coriander, think of its Samurai-like qualities, ask it to instruct you in its sense of rhythm, its strength. A colour I often visualize with it is a deep magenta, which can give a well-rounded sense of attunement – you might like to feel that radiating around you. This is especially useful if you are trying to make a decision and your mind is wandering over all the possibilities.

One step at a time.

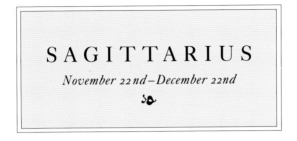

SAGITTARIUS

November 22nd–December 22nd

The three months of WINTER are called the period of closing and storing. Water freezes and the Earth cracks open. One should not disturb one's Yang...The pulse is that of the kidneys.

Nei Ching

In winter body energy goes inwards and should be conserved. To the Chinese the Yang, or active force, is naturally dormant, giving way to the Yin or stored, inherent energy.

SAGITTARIUS NEW MOON: THANKSGIVING MOON

Scorpio tested us, forced us into a necessary retreat. Now, as we enter the generous sign of Sagittarius, we have the chance to reflect, give thanks and prepare for the winter celebrations. But this sign brings the snow and ice and warmth no longer comes from the environment, so we should look for steady, reliable sources of heat.

The organs responsible for preserving body energy are believed to be the kidneys. Damp winter days often bring pain and stiffness, especially in the back. Good, sustaining nourishment for the kidneys comes mainly from roots, nuts, beans and grain, foods which conserve the radiance of the summer sun and were once the major part of a winter diet. One essence that the kidneys really love is Ginger.

GINGER (*Zingiber officinale*)

Ginger root is a natural storekeeper. Under the old 'doctrine of signatures'[*] its shape shows a special affinity for the human digestive system. This great friend to mankind will stimulate the flow of digestive juices, reduce excessive moisture, ease pain and raise body temperature.

> Extreme fear is injurious to the kidneys, but fear can be overcome by contemplation.
>
> *Nei Ching*

The smell of fear can linger in winter as people find it difficult to cope with the restricting effect of the cold. Ginger's warmth and courage understands vulnerability, particularly when it is disguised by bravado. Anyone who is putting on this kind of act will sooner or later suffer from a depletion of energy. The sustaining nature of ginger is an excellent remedy to gently release emotions that have been locked up by a lack of trust.

[*] Doctrine of Signatures: the relationship between the shape of a plant and the corresponding human body organ

The rich, familiar smell of this gentle friend reminds me of the forthcoming festive season and that alone produces a feeling of wellbeing.

GINGER: MEDITATION

It is easy to feel that the work our bodies do is not really a part of US. We damage them by ignoring nature's basic laws and also by deep and prolonged anxieties which can act as a poison, eventually having an effect at a cellular level.

Put a few drops of ginger in a burner and sit somewhere warm and comfortable in a dimly-lit room. Place your hands together between your navel and diaphragm.

Breathe gently for a few minutes, inhaling the ginger and feel its warmth circulating, especially around the kidneys and lower half of the body. Regulate your breathing to a slower and more even pace, raising your chest as you breathe in and dropping it gently as you breathe out.

Allow the warmth of the ginger to nourish your stomach, feel it growing stronger, stronger. Do this for a minute or two and then move your hands to below the navel and visualize the energy circulating through the lower digestive organs. Allow the ginger to give them a sense of stability. Now move your hands around to your kidneys and do the same. Thank them for all their hard work and allow the ginger to protect their vital energy.

Bring your hands back to their original position.

Breathe in: Draw in the nourishment of the ginger.

Breathe out: Breathe out deep seated fears.

Do this for about five minutes and when you have finished thank your body for nourishing you. Regular use of this meditation will help you feel more at one with your bodily functions.

I trust my body.

SAGITTARIUS FULL MOON: MOON OF PURE PERCEPTION

Now Earth's energy is reaching for the crown, point of union with the divine force.

ANGELICA (*Angelica archangelica*)

> ...therefore some call this an herb of the Holy Ghost; others more moderate called it Angelica, because of its angelical virtues, and that name it retains still, and all nations follow it so near as their dialect will permit.

> Nicholas Culpeper, *The English Physician*, 1653

People have often dedicated herbs to their gods if they possessed outstanding healing properties. Angelica has a reputation as an elixir and saviour for the entire system and is said to have been sought by the

East in much the same way as Ginseng has migrated West. In folklore its associations with magic and superstition emphasize the fine line between what manifests as good or evil. Like Coriander it is from the Parsley family – and remember, Hemlock, the poisoner, is a cousin and resembles it in appearance. Both plants are often suffused with the same healing purple.

This plant loves high, wet woods and cool, damp places. Immensely tall and striking, its large hollow stems attract poisons from the earth and evaporate them into the atmosphere. This action is mirrored in its effect on the psyche. A true exorcist, it draws out fears, phobias, timidity, indecision and replaces them with a sense of reality and deep relaxation.

The term 'angelic' evokes something fragile and illusive, but this belies its true meaning. The bible always refers to angels as fiery beings surrounded by coals of fire, crystalline forms, sapphires and quartzes, with 'legs of burnished brass'. Beings who confront rather than manifest quietly. Angelica is like that, it belongs to the Sun and its fiery essence directs a current of vital energy into your soul.

And from the gate thrown open issued beaming
A beautiful and mighty Thing of Light,
Radiant with glory, like a banner streaming
Victorious with some world o'er-throwing fight. . .

Lord Byron, 'The Archangel', 19th Century

In Greek *angelos* means messenger. We are in Advent, the time of the Annunciation, when the Angel Gabriel brought his extraordinary message to Mary. The sensation of an angelic presence is sometimes registered momentarily by extremely sensitive people when they inhale Angelica. For the merest fraction of a second, that fine curtain between the Truth and what we perceive to be true can be lifted by such a powerful fragrance.

Angelica's scent is not beautiful, but it encourages one to question. It is a bit like life. Overpowering sometimes, at others wonderfully refreshing. It is hard to describe, but within it there is a single note that touches a higher level of being. Like a tiny bell, an angelus, softly calling, it asks us 'what do you really believe in?'

If applied to the skin, Angelica has the potential for photosensitivity.

ANGELICA: MEDITATION

Do not burn or diffuse Angelica, simply put a drop on a smelling strip and inhale it every now and then. Its effect can be like a mirror, so you may like to use this as a visual aid.

Inhale the scent. Then put the smelling strip down, but keep the fragrance in your consciousness. Angelica has a very distinctive aroma and once you get used to it, you will be able to do this.

Visualize a mirror: it is cloudy as if someone has breathed on it. Gradually it clears. In it is the reflection of someone rather beautiful, but you can't make out who it is, is it a man or a woman? The person in the reflection is holding up another mirror to you. That one is also cloudy. When it clears, who will you recognize?

*W*INTER SOLSTICE:
DECEMBER 21ST SHORTEST DAY

A lamp are you, above all stars of night, to guide sailors in the dusk; lovely is your colour, sweet maid, standing in the doorway of the Pole.

Carnelian, 'The Pole Star: An Epigram', 19th Century

The sun is at its lowest point in the sky, Darkness has triumphed over Light. Trees are bare, days are short and nights long. Shadows linger on the cold, frozen ground. Only the constancy of the Moon's influence remains and underground her magnetism is already stirring a new cycle of life.

On this day and this day only, prehistoric high altars still reflect the rays of the rising sun. On this, our oldest festival, early man directed all his energy into calling back the Light. Fires, feasts and candles at Christmas are a reminder of an ancient and primeval desire.

From now until Twelfth Night, we enter a period of mystic symbolism, inhabited by the Yule Log – the wheel of life; the Christmas Tree – the tree of life; mistletoe – union of sun and moon; The Holly and the Ivy: evergreen symbols of rebirth; and many others, including of course, Gold, Frankincense and Myrrh.

> And he shall put the incense upon the fire before the
> Lord that the cloud of the incense may cover the mercy
> seat that is upon the testimony, that he die not.
>
> Leviticus 16:13

FRANKINCENSE (*Boswellia carteri* – and other species)
The purifying smoke of Frankincense has linked believers with unseen
worlds for millennia. Balls of it were found in Tutankhamun's tomb
and, like Myrrh, it had a vital role to play in the burial of priest-kings.

> Who is this that cometh out of the wilderness like pillars
> of smoke, perfumed with myrrh and frankincense, with
> all the powders of the merchant?   Song of Solomon 3:6

Like Myrrh, Frankincense is a desert tree. Its family name means 'Dry
Fire' and its oozing resin releases a delicate blue transparency that
absorbs the intense rays of the sun as they strike the desert rocks. The
spicy, balsamic scent has an uplifting quality that gives it light. In a
fragrance burner on a cold winter's day it will infuse the atmosphere
with the pure fire of the desert air.

The desert is a place of extremes. All its creatures must be able
to withstand the intense heat of the day and penetrating cold of
night. Their resilience is matched only by their counterparts in arctic
regions. Such places have a unique beauty and are alive with a
cosmic activity that is surely transcendental – no wonder mystics

sought refuge there among the sacred plants.

The power of Frankincense is to burn off the surface of the unknown. Called an auric cleanser, it will clear the mirror through which we view our lives, creating a channel between past, present and future. Its action is to alter the way we perceive past experiences without destroying that vital link in the understanding of the forces that shape our lives.

This generous essence gives us a choice. We can bask in its protective aura, or rekindle our inner fire with a new sense or purpose – both are on offer. Inhaling it brings a sensation of deeply penetrating warmth. It is extremely beneficial to breathing, bringing a deeper and slower rhythm and is an effective aid for meditation.

Use it in cold situations where weakness and death prevail, if you have undergone a deeply emotional experience, or if you are bereaved. Use it especially if you are hanging onto dismal thoughts associated with the past, or simply if you wish to enter a higher sphere.

Like all powerful fragrances, Frankincense must be treated with the utmost respect. Its message is that the universal force moves only forward. In reality there is no going back and there is freedom in that.

FRANKINCENSE: MEDITATION

Put a few drops of Frankincense in a fragrance burner above the hearth on a cold winter's night, or by the radiator if you do not have an open fire.

Light a candle. Sit quietly looking at the candle glow and breathe deeply and slowly for about five minutes. The rich fragrance of

Frankincense will fill the room.

Through the window the sky may seem black, but it is not, it is a deep indigo. The blue-black of indigo plumbs hidden depths and is the great regenerator. Think of the sky as it enfolds the earth and remember this.

Now close your eyes. Continue to breathe deeply and regularly. If you have just lost a loved one, remember that they, too, are part of this cycle. Say their name a few times and wish them well on their journey.

Tomorrow I begin again.

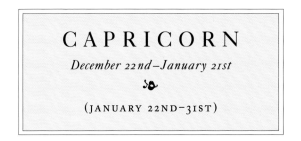

CAPRICORN

December 22nd–January 21st

(JANUARY 22ND–31ST)

The year has come full circle. As the old Sagittarian moon wanes Capricorn returns to cover the land with ice and snow. Its solid, stabilizing influence is reflected in the beautiful, deep green of the Pine, impressive now, against a pure, white background. This was the tree the Druids chose for 22nd December, the first day of their waxing year.

CAPRICORN NEW MOON: FROZEN WISHES MOON

> And out of the ground made the Lord God to grow every tree that is pleasant to the sight, and good for food; the tree of life also in the midst of the garden, and the tree of knowledge of good and evil. Genesis II:9

PINE NEEDLE (*Pinus sylvestris* – and other species)
The towering Pine tree was a link between heaven and earth. With

deeply penetrating roots and branches reaching to the sky, its spiritual stature rivalled the Oak and its rich sāp was thought to stimulate growth in everything. This immortal 'Tree of Life' appears in almost every religion and culture and has become our Christmas Tree.

Pine trees love a high mountainside in the northern hemisphere where the air is clear. They live with little sun and freezing temperatures, yet there is nothing dreary about their lives. A natural pine forest is bathed in luminous green glass radiance as it reflects back the light through its shimmering needles. In winter there is a sense of the mystic, like the inside of a cathedral, but in summer it is pungent and alive with cosmic energy as the trees generate heat to sustain them through the cold months.

To inhale essence of Pine is to direct a current of energy into the senses and imbibe fresh, clean mountain air. This tree loves to *breathe* and it allows us to do so too. In winter a fresh supply of oxygen is vital for every cell.

The Tree of Life is an archetype and is invariably shown with fruits, colours or sacred lights. The planets and stars, the colours of the spectrum, these are the lights on the Christmas Tree. Pine shows us the unity of these elements in a dignified, harmonious whole, it is the supreme balancer.

From this powerful symbol we can learn many things. Pine speaks of social stability, self-worth and endurance, and can help us to understand why we have chosen our own particular path. Use it to gain an understanding of your place in the universal scheme.

PINE: MEDITATION

> A beautiful pine makes music to me, it is not hired;
> through Christ, I fare no worse at any time than you do.
>
> Irish, anon, 'The Hermit's Hut', 10th Century

Put a few drops of Pine in a fragrance burner and light the flame.

Sit comfortably and close your eyes. Visualize the green pine tree rising like a pole out of the white snow.

Along it are arranged the seven rainbow colours, Red at the base, Violet at top. Now imagine another tree as the central pole running through your own body. Arrange the colours against it: Red at the base; Orange in the small of the back; Yellow in the middle; Green between the shoulders; Blue at the base of the skull; Indigo in the forehead; Violet right on top of the head.[*] Now you match the tree. Feel rooted in the earth – and stretch out your arms as the branches reach up to the sky. Keep your spine straight, but at rest. Feel suspended in time.

Relax your arms and breathe in the fragrance of Pine, lifting your chest with the intake of each breath, then gently relaxing it.

Breathe in:	See a star at the top of the tree, radiating a bright, white light.
Breathe in and out gently:	Watch that white light flow downwards through the colours, each one in turn.

---

[*] If you cannot visualize the colours, imagine the radiant green of the tree against the white snow.

As the tree is bathed in light, let the scent of Pine become a current running through you.

Breathe out: Allow the colours to dissolve and then let the tree fade away too, leaving only the cosmic white light.

I am a child of the universe.

CHRISTMAS DAY:
25TH DECEMBER

The modest Rose puts forth a thorn,
The humble sheep a threat'ning horn;
While the lilly white shall in Love delight,
Nor a thorn, nor a threat, stain her beauty bright.

William Blake, 'The Lilly', 18th Century

THE MADONNA LILY

It is said that the Lily will die in the shadow of the Rose. This may be true, it dislikes artificial environments or crowded places.

The Rose has given itself to be fussed over in the material world, but the Lily is still set apart and has changed little. Rose delights our gardens with a myriad of scents and colours, but Lily floats its fragile fragrance over wasteland and high rocky slopes.

Paintings of the Madonna and Child favour the Rose, but those of the Annunciation often show Gabriel holding a white Madonna Lily in his hand.

If the five-petalled Rose shows us heaven on earth, the six-petalled Lily speaks of earth as it is in heaven.

To my knowledge there is as yet no natural essence of Lily available commercially.

Perhaps we are not yet ready to receive it.

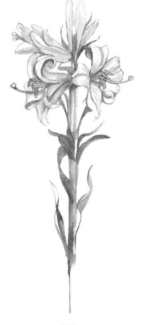

BIBLIOGRAPHY

A Celtic Miscellany, trans. Kenneth Hurlston Jackson, Routledge and Kegan Paul, 1951

The Essene Gospel of Peace, Book Two, Edmond Bordeaux Szekely, I.B.S. Internacional, Box 205, Matsqui, British Columbia, Canada VOX ISO

Tao To Ching, trans. Gia-Fu Feng and Jane English, Gower Publishing Co. Ltd. 1973

The Yellow Emperor's Classic of Internal Medicine, trans. Ilza Veith, University of California Press, 1949

Touch the Earth: A Self-Portrait of Indian Existence, ed. T.C. McLuhan, Garnstone Press Ltd, 1972

FURTHER READING

Robert Tisserand, *The Art of Aromatherapy*, CW Daniel, 1977

Scott Cunningham, *Magical Aromatherapy*, Llewellyn, 1989

Patricia Davis, *Subtle Aromatherapy*, CW Daniel, 1991

Vicky Wall, *The Miracle of Colour Healing*, The Aquarian Press, 1990

Steve Van Toller and George H. Dodd, *Perfumery, The Psychology and Biology of Fragrance*, Chapman & Hall 1988

৵৹ UNITED KINGDOM

A list of aromatherapy associations, therapists and reputable suppliers can be obtained from:

Aromatherapy Organisations Council
Wesley House
Stockwell Head
Hinckley
Leicestershire
LE10 1RD

OTHER USEFUL ADDRESSES

Aromatherapy Quarterly
5 Ranelagh Avenue
London
SW13 0BY

Aromatherapy Times
Journal of the International
    Federation of Aromatherapists
Department of Continuing
    Education
The Royal Masonic Hospital
Ravenscourt Park
London
W6 0TN

International Journal of Aromatherapy
PO Box 746
Hove
East Sussex
BN3 3XA

Aromatherapy World
41 Leicester Road
Hinckley
Leicestershire
LE10 1 LW

AUSTRALIA

Auroma
Australian Botanical Products Pty Ltd
39 Melverton Drive
Hallam
Victoria 3803

Springfields
Suite 2, 1 Johnston Lane
Lane Cove
Sydney

Sunspirit Oils Pty Ltd
PO Box 85
Byron Bay
NSW 2481

Oleum Aromatherapy
Modern Skin Care Pty Ltd
175 Newcastle Street
Fyshwick
ACT 2609

OTHER USEFUL ADDRESSES

Simply Essential
Magazine of the Australian Branch of
  the International Federation of
  Aromatherapists
24 Morgan Street
Kingsgrove
NSW 2208

USA

Aroma Vera Inc
33844 So. Robertson Place
Los Angeles
CA 90034

Ledet Oils
PO Box 2354
Fair Oaks
CA 95628

OTHER USEFUL ADDRESSES

Common Scents
The American Aromatherapy
  Association
PO Box 3679
South Pasadena
CA 91031
Telephone: 818 457 1742
Fax: 818 300 8099

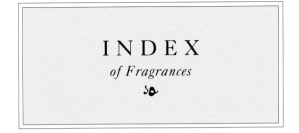

INDEX
of Fragrances